MORE ADVICE FROM THE BACK DOCTOR

HAMILTON HALL M.D.

MORE ADVICE FROM THE BACK DOCTOR

M&S

Canadian Cataloguing in Publication Data

Hall, Hamilton, 1938–
  More advice from the back doctor

Includes index.

ISBN 0-7710-3771-6

1. Back – Care and hygiene. 2. Backache. I. Title.

RD768.H36 1987   617′.56   C87-093294-2

Printed and bound in Canada

Design by Esther Pflug
Anatomical illustrations © Margot Mackay, ANSCAD, BSc, AAM
Other illustrations © Peter Honor

This book is not intended to replace the services of a physician. Any application of the recommendations set forth in the following pages is at the reader's discretion and sole risk.

The Canadian Publishers
McClelland and Stewart
481 University Avenue
Toronto M5G 2E9

CONTENTS

INTRODUCTION

Eight years ago, I set out to write my first book, *The Back Doctor*, realizing there were countless numbers of people out there who needed information to help them overcome back pain. I expected to reach a lot of them, but I never dreamed my message would travel virtually around the world.

I got the first inkling of the book's wide acceptance when publishers in Britain and Australia joined with those in Canada and the United States to produce the initial editions. Next, other publishers translated my words into French, Hebrew, and Dutch (in The Netherlands I am now proud to be known as De Rugdokter).

But the most delightful evidence of a world-girdling interest in my message came to me in a personal letter. The writer was Dr. Jay Keystone, an acquaintance of mine during our days as resident physicians in Toronto. Since my field was orthopedic surgery and Jay's was tropical medicine, our differing schedules set us on diverging paths. Over the years I lost touch with him and had no idea that he'd developed a bad back. All that changed in 1983, when I received his one-page letter from Hyderabad, India. Jay explained he was on a sabbatical studying leprosy and was writing in haste to describe an experience he felt was just too good to keep to himself. His letter went on:

Yesterday I was invited to meet an octogenarian Anglo-Indian retired school principal who lives not far from my hotel. She was the friend of a missionary and also of the British physician under whom I am studying in Hyderabad.

I was taken to the back of a rather run-down school where several small hotel-like rooms were located. Here, we found a little old Indian lady whose mental faculties were very well preserved. She sat in a darkened room, surrounded by her belongings, which were rather meager.

After a round of tea and biscuits the conversation turned to my painful back, which has worsened as a consequence of riding along bumpy roads in three-wheeled "auto-rickshaws." I could hardly believe my eyes when from under a pile of dust-covered books she pulled out a copy of *The Back Doctor*. I am now reading your book, which I was unable to find at several Toronto book stores because they ran out of stock!

By the time I sat down to begin this sequel, I was convinced not only that I had found a huge audience for my message but also that there was no shortage of fresh material of potentially wide interest. It's true that when friends and patients heard I was working on a second book, many wanted to know, "What could you possibly write that isn't already in your first book?" But for every reader who evidently regarded *The Back Doctor* as *the* complete book of its kind, there was another who told me, "The things you wrote were helpful, but I wish you'd said more about such-and-such."

And so, as well as introducing new topics, I have responded to many requests for information on subjects I dealt with only fleetingly in *The Back Doctor*.

Patients faced with the prospect of back surgery wanted more information on the nature of their operations and additional tips on the art of post-operative recovery. I have obliged. Other readers wanted me to elaborate on neck pain, a common complaint that deserves the full discussion found here. A number of people were concerned about the effects of back pain on sexual relations and pregnancy, and many were hesitant to broach the subject with their doctors. I have tried to address their concerns. Our knowledge of the chronic pain syndrome – a sadly misunderstood behavioral disease that too often afflicts back patients – has advanced so remarkably that I felt it would be useful to describe the condition in detail. And so, in thinking through the scope of the new book, I assigned each of these subjects a chapter of its own.

I also felt an obligation to respond to increasing concern over two widely discussed conditions that create back pain: osteoporosis, a sometimes troublesome aspect of the aging process; and spinal stenosis, about which surgeons have learned much since publication of *The Back Doctor*. (In fact, spinal stenosis has emerged as such a significant problem in my practice that I have revised my classification of the causes of common backache to include it as Type Four.)

The very nature of this demand for information suggested a format for the new book: why not assemble all the questions patients kept asking me, add a few questions I sometimes wish they *would* ask, and then provide my answers? Although I did not foresee what a comfortable choice it would prove to be, the more I worked with this question-and-answer approach, the better I liked it. It lends itself readily to the informal, conversational style that I favor when working with my patients. And I hope readers will feel, as I do, that it has enabled me to put across much useful information, including some fairly technical concepts, in a clear and meaningful way.

One additional point of style: like many other writers these days, I wish there were a singular pronoun in English, equivalent to "he" or "she," to refer to a person of either sex. I got around the problem in most cases by using such neutral words as "you" and "the patient." In a few instances, I resorted, reluctantly, to the clumsy he-or-she construction. But where those alternatives weren't workable, I simply said "he" – trusting my readers to realize that, where the context allowed, the one pronoun was intended to mean either a male or a female.

I must confess that the prospect of writing a second book presented several opportunities I found attractive for personal reasons. It would provide a chance to convey my enthusiasm for technological advances that represent good news for patients and doctors alike. (I am as enthusiastic about an emerging diagnostic tool called magnetic resonance imaging as I was about the invaluable CT scan when I wrote *The Back Doctor*.) A second book would enable me, as well, to bring readers up to date on my evolving concepts of back care, such as my increased appreciation for the therapeutic value of extension exercises. And it could serve as a platform from which to express my growing concern over the way personal injury lawsuits are discouraging some back patients from getting well.

In a new book I could also report the latest findings and developments at the Canadian Back Institute. This last possibility proved to be even more timely than I anticipated. While this book was going through the writing process, the Institute went through an exciting new stage in its evolution. The CBI had a modest beginning in 1974, as a series of informal lectures intended to help small groups of my own patients with their back problems. In its first metamorphosis, it developed into the Canadian Back Education Units, with branches in several Canadian provinces and U.S. states and an outpost in Perth, Australia.

Even after it adopted its present name and embarked on several research projects, the institute for several years remained essentially an educational organization. Then, less than two years ago, to fill the gap between the treatment it recommended and the treatment most patients received, the CBI broadened its scope significantly to become a comprehensive center for education, assessment, treatment, and training, employing modern techniques of non-invasive therapy while conducting research into the value of specific exercises for the various types of back pain. In the course of its research, the CBI, at last count, had studied and analyzed the problems and progress of more than 15,000 victims of common backache.

Now, encouraged by the favorable response of patients within reach of its charter headquarters, the new-style CBI is expanding to other locations, with every expectation of becoming a continent-wide operation by the early 1990s.

From the moment I first considered writing a second book, I realized that its fundamental message would have to be identical to that of *The Back Doctor*. After all, although my approach to back problems continues to evolve, my basic beliefs remain unchanged. In fact, CBI studies have now confirmed opinions I adopted years ago as simple, self-evident truths: that the more you know about your back, the better able you are to care for it, and that taking the responsibility for your own recovery helps guarantee a good result. I make no apology for restating these and other essential principles, but I have tried to present my ideas in a fresh and timely fashion, to reinforce what readers of *The Back Doctor* already know, while providing the essential information to others.

With the publication of my first book, some people formed the erroneous opinion that in prescribing exercises for the relief of back pain, I favored quite a different approach than that of my good friend Robin McKenzie. A physical therapist from New Zealand, Robin has worked with unfailing energy to demonstrate the value of a therapy program tailored to the patient's specific requirements. And more than any other person I am aware of, Robin has been instrumental in re-establishing the importance of extension exercising – an achievement I am happy to acknowledge. After reading this sequel, anyone familiar with Robin McKenzie's work should realize that there never has been any professional conflict between us.

Only time and my readers' responses will tell whether I have succeeded in creating the book I intended. If I have, some of the credit must certainly go to several individuals.

I am indebted to Tony Melles, senior physiotherapist and director of the Canadian Back Institute, and to the rest of its staff, whose contributions to the development of the CBI exercise program are reflected extensively in this book.

My discussion of the chronic pain syndrome owes much to the special expertise of Allan Walton, Dr. Rickey Miller, and Dr. David Corey, whose diligent work in this previously neglected area of human psychology continues to shed welcome light on a difficult problem.

The section on osteoporosis was prepared with the generous help of Dr. William Sturtridge, whose knowledge and experience as a specialist in metabolic bone disease and whose ability to speak intelligibly to a surgical confrere form a rare and invaluable combination.

Without the perseverance and gentle pressure of Hal Tennant, this book would never have been written. I welcome this opportunity to declare publicly how much I have learned from our long association about the vicissitudes of the English language and the subtleties of the writer's art. Hal has become more than a genial collaborator; he is a valued friend.

I am delighted that Peter Honor agreed to illustrate this text. I have used his pictures in my talks for years, to rave reviews. I always remember hearing from a doctor in California who wrote asking not for a copy of a speech I had delivered there but for copies of the cartoons I'd used!

A word of thanks to the Colberts, Nancy, Stanley, and David, whose expert guidance and sound advice have done so much to enlighten me on the ways of the publishing world.

Finally, I acknowledge the help and support of Ellen Seligman. As my current editor and my former back patient, she holds a unique perspective. Her professional insight and personal empathy have touched every chapter of this book.

Hamilton Hall, M.D., F.R.C.S. (C)
Toronto
November 1986

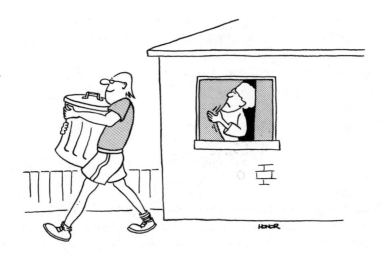

1. HAVE YOU HUGGED YOUR GARBAGE CAN TODAY?

No matter how many doctors or therapists you may see, or how many treatments or operations you may have, the basic responsibility for your back and its care rests with you.

You have a choice. You can allow your back to rule your life by influencing your every decision, however big or small. Or you can devise a strategy for taking charge, so that *you*, not your back pain, will determine how you live and what you do with your life.

Once you have resolved to take control, the trick is to pursue your strategy with single-minded determination – yet not allow it to become an obsession. The distinction between the two is not that hard to make if your intentions are clear and honest and your strategy is sound.

I can think of two patients whose attitudes readily illustrate the difference. One patient was a woman in her late forties who had been coming to me with a back problem for years. Originally an active person, she had developed the unfortunate habit of dwelling constantly on her back pain. As an ardent traveler, for instance, she would dramatize her suffering by hiring ambulances to take her to and from airports.

On one of her visits to me, I conducted my routine tests and found that her back had undergone significant improvement since the last time I'd seen her. But, as inclined as ever to accentuate the negative, she didn't see it that way.

"What are you doing these days?" I asked.

"Nothing," she said. "I've even given up grocery shopping. I can't lift the heavy bags."

I asked why she didn't have someone else carry her groceries out to her car.

"Well," she said, "I'd still have to unload them when I got home."

Of course she could have gotten help from a family member or neighbor or could have unpacked the bags an item at a time.

I'd forgotten how fond this woman was of the Yes-But game, and how skilled she was at rejecting any positive thought that might be expressed about her condition. Despite my many attempts to provide her with reassurance and constructive advice, she had remained determined to dwell on her problem and defy anyone to help her get better. I realized there was no point in making more suggestions; there is little a doctor can do or say when a person refuses to be helped.

Apart from back pain, her determination was about the only thing that woman had in common with another patient whose experience was related to me by a colleague. At the age of twenty-three, in a careless plunge into the shallow end of a swimming pool, Richard crushed three vertebrae in the thoracic, or middle, section of his spine. Fortunately there was no damage to the spinal cord.

After a short stay in the hospital, he visited several doctors, each of whom told him the same thing: although the fractures had created an obvious and painful bump on his back, there was nothing anyone could do for him. He simply had to get on with his life as best he could.

Unemployed, Richard went looking for work – *any* kind of work. But prospective employers turned him down, time and again, because of his back. Fed up with rejection, he got into an exercise program and began strengthening the uninjured parts of his back, so that they could take the load and ease the strain on those deformed vertebrae. After several months he got to the point where he could control the discomfort – but he still couldn't land a job.

Finally, he went into yet another job interview – with a new tactic: when he was asked whether he had any medical problems, he lied. He declared that his health was perfect. He never mentioned his back. The company hired him and sent him for a routine physical check-up. Since the slight deformity from the old fractures was still visible, he feared the jig was up. But in the examining room, Richard struck up a conversation about fitness and exercise and got the doctor so engrossed that the man never did get around to looking at Richard's back. Richard passed the medical, started work, and is now considered a valuable employee.

While I can't condone his lie, Richard's attitude offers a refreshing contrast to the Yes-But responses I heard from the other patient, and clearly illustrates the important part that positive thinking can play in overcoming even the most serious back problem.

You have often said publicly that roughly four out of five people in this part of the world will suffer from common backache at some time in their lives. Does that mean back pain is inevitable for most people?

Not at all. A great many people could avoid some or all of that pain if they practiced certain exercises regularly and adopted better habits in the course of their daily living.

Are you saying that most people abuse their backs without realizing it?

They do, in the sense that they place unnecessary strain on their spines, either without realizing it or at least without knowing how to avoid it. In their everyday activities, most people constantly subject their backs to many minor loads. These strains, combined with the natural wear and tear of aging, lead to back pain.

When the spine ages, the small joints connecting the vertebrae lose their smooth lining, and the roughened surfaces rub together. The discs become less resilient and bulge out between the bones, sometimes pressing on a nerve. Any of these conditions can produce severe, even excruciating, pain. In its early stages, however, this wear and tear is so gradual that most people are unaware of it. Then, one day, a person may unwittingly place a little more stress on the back than those worn parts of the spine can handle –

an unaccustomed twist of the trunk, for instance, or an attempt at an unusually heavy lift – and the result is a sort of "last straw" effect. That's when your spine will send you a clear message – in the form of a sudden attack of pain.

And I suppose the worse the wear has been up to that moment, the more painful the attack will be.

Oddly enough, that's not so. The amount of pain often has little relationship to the seriousness of the problem. You can suffer a lot of pain from a back condition that is in fact just a minor sprain on a vertebral joint, just as you can feel a great deal of pain from whacking your funnybone without actually damaging your arm.

At the other end of the scale, I've seen serious conditions, such as sustained pressure on a nerve, causing muscle weakness, that produced very little pain.

But you say people could avoid many of those painful attacks by adopting better living habits.

Certainly. The ways you stand, walk, sit, lie down, sleep, work, play, and go about all the other routine things you do every day, control how much load your spine must endure and whether a worn joint or disc will suddenly produce new pain.

And that's what you're referring to when you talk about having a strategy against backache. Can you suggest a standard set of rules?

I don't believe in uniform rules for everyone, because something that works well for one person may not work for another. It's better to develop an individual strategy based on a few general principles.

What are the general principles of good back care?

Apart from proper exercise and ordinary common sense about the things you expect your back to do, the one basic principle I like to cite is summed up in a phrase that was popular in the 1960s: "If it feels good, do it." If some position you use in standing or sitting or working makes your back feel good, it's the right position for you. It certainly won't cause trouble, and it probably reduces the load on your back.

Is the opposite true? If some activity hurts your back, is it harming your spine?

Probably not harming, in the sense of causing damage. It may hurt a little, or even a lot, because it's aggravating a sore spot, but it's unlikely to be causing physical injury. When you feel pain, your back isn't necessarily saying, "This is damaging me." More likely, it's saying, "Look out! You're making me do something I don't want to do." Even if you were in perfect condition, you'd get a similar message from various parts of your body if you ran the Boston Marathon or swam the English Channel. Tender though it may be, your back is far too tough to be harmed – that is, damaged – by a little extra exertion.

There may be times when you will consider it worthwhile to ignore that message from your spine and put up with a little extra pain to get on with your daily work or to carry on with some activity you particularly enjoy, like golfing. Or making love.

Of course there will be a great many more occasions when you will want to avoid pain because there is nothing to be gained by putting up with it and there's a lot to be gained by adopting the habits that make your back feel good.

That brings me to a more specific question: my back hurts when I wake up in the morning. Do you think I need a better mattress?

Possibly but not necessarily. The most important consideration is your sleeping position. I'd suggest sleeping on your back with a fat pillow under your knees, or on your side with your legs tucked up and a large pillow between your thighs. Experiment. Any position that makes you comfortable and prevents your back from aching in the morning is a good position for you.

What about sleeping on my stomach?

Generally speaking, you are better off not sleeping on your stomach. When you do, your back arches, squeezing the spinal joints together and often causing pain. However, if you've always found that position comfortable and it's the only way you can get a decent night's sleep, then it would be foolish to change. I'd suggest, though, that you try putting a thin pillow under your pelvis. This will modify the arch in your back and reduce the pressure on the small joints.

But don't a lot of people fall asleep in one position and wake up in another? And maybe sleep in a lot of other positions between times? I know I do.

Of course. And it can be one of those situations where you're damned if you do and damned if you don't. It's true that during sleep you may assume certain positions that will aggravate a bad back. On the other hand, a certain amount of shifting around is good for you. Sleeping in the same position for hours at a time may lead to temporary but painful stiffness of the joints in the morning.

If you make a point of it, you can train yourself to assume or avoid almost any position – just as we all train ourselves, from early childhood, not to fall out of bed while we're sleeping.

What if I sleep in my most comfortable position and still wake up with back pain?

In that case, your mattress could be to blame. If it sags, or is resting on a sagging base, it's probably not providing the support you need.

How much support does my back need? Should I consider putting a board under the mattress?

The right amount of firmness is a matter of personal preference. If a mattress feels right when you lie on it and lets you turn over without difficulty or discomfort, it's right for you. If you have a sleeping partner who is much heavier than you are, you might be more comfortable with an extra-firm mattress or one constructed with individual-acting coils to prevent a "trough" that keeps you sliding downhill.

As for the old board-under-the-mattress idea, that's passé – a relic of the time before the modern box-spring was in common use, when mattresses were generally supported on a sagging link-spring base. A board on a good box-spring won't make much difference, and if you put a board on top of the mattress, why bother with a mattress at all? You might as well just sleep on the board – or on the bare floor.

Would it be a good idea to switch to a waterbed?

A waterbed, particularly a heated one, is designed to help you relax and avoid the restlessness you were talking about a minute ago. Many people find a waterbed helpful since it provides full, contour support for the spine and reduces movement during sleep. Others say it makes their backs feel worse. I suspect that's because they change position so infrequently that their back joints become stiff. And so, again, it's a matter of individual choice. Rather than make the purchase and risk disappointment, why not try one out for a few nights? You may find a waterbed store that offers a money-back trial, or if you're planning a trip, you could look for a hotel or motel that has waterbeds. Or maybe you can stay with a friend who owns one.

What about lying in a hammock?

If you have back pain, I'd suggest limiting your time in a hammock to a couple of hours. Otherwise, you're likely to have trouble, for two reasons. First, it's impossible to lie in a hammock and maintain the normal curvature in your low back; there is no uniform support. And second, a hammock doesn't allow you to move around to avoid continuous pressure on the same part of your spine. If you try to roll over, the hammock rolls with you. That's the great appeal: the swaying action offers a sort of return-to-the-womb feeling. But it's hard on your back.

Sometimes in the morning my neck, especially, seems stiff. Would a special pillow help?

It's certainly worth a try. Your neck has a particular problem whenever you sleep on your side: with your head on the pillow and your shoulder on the mattress, your neck is often tilted to one side. Worse still, it is suspended, unsupported, like a clothesline between its two end poles. Naturally, it sags, and that increases the pressure on one side of the cervical spine. Attempts to avoid that sag have given rise to the design of special cervical pillows to ease the pressure on the neck. One popular type is known as the butterfly pillow because of its shape. You lie with your neck over the "body" of the butterfly, and as long as you remain that way, the "wings" on each side provide the stability you need to keep your head in the right position.

Other pillows, more elegant, are designed in shapes based on biomechanical studies, but their purpose is the same as that of the butterfly. Some of these give you support for the head as well as for the neck. Others are designed so that you can roll over.

Like everything else, these pillows have their enthusiasts and their detractors. In some cases, even the designers admit their pillows will seem uncomfortable at first. And this raises another point: some of these items are expensive, as pillows go, and only you can decide whether they're worth the money.

If waterbeds and special pillows are sometimes helpful at night, what about using various supports and aids during the day?

Back supports, foot-rests, and various other devices can provide temporary relief from back pain – and I'm all for that. But it's important to realize these aids are *passive* ways of achieving temporary relief, not substitutes for an active program of regular back care and exercise.

I saw someone with a portable folding foot-rest. What do you think of carrying something like that?

The principle is fine, although personally I wouldn't bother with one of those gadgets. They're like many safety devices that sound great in theory but seldom get used. However, if you like the idea of a portable foot-rest, and you're willing to spend the money on it, there's no reason why you shouldn't own one. But I've always been willing to take my chances on finding a low rail or step – whatever's handy.

What about posture? Are there certain habits you should adopt?

Yes, there are. You should begin by recognizing that your spine has a natural, moderate curvature that doesn't take kindly to extremes. Your back isn't comfortable when it's ramrod straight or when that natural contour is exaggerated.

Then how *would* you describe the best posture for standing?

Try to position your body directly under your head and neck. In an easy and relaxed manner settle your head in line with your shoulders, then gently tuck in your buttocks to tilt the top of your pelvis backward and reduce any excess curve in your lower spine. The effect should be one of standing up straight without strain. To further avoid discomfort while standing, change your position frequently to vary the pressure on all parts of your back.

From gym class I remember a posture called the "monkey slump," which relaxed our backs. Would that achieve the same thing?

No, the posture I am suggesting will leave you in no danger of being mistaken for an ape in the zoo. By all means do yourself a favor once in a while by standing in a slump for a few minutes, with your head and shoulders well forward and your arms dangling down. You'll find that stance relaxing because it stretches out the muscles in the upper back and reduces any excess curve in the lower spine. But it's not good as a regular form of posture. Besides looking silly, it creates a whole new pattern of increased load on the spine.

With proper posture, you're relaxing without actually slumping. You'll know, from the feeling of comfort, when you've got it right – especially if you have Type One back pain, which originates from pressure on worn joints. If you are overweight, you probably have a tendency to arch your back too much, and the strain-free posture will help relieve your pain.

Another elementary technique to reduce an excessive curve in your low back is to avoid standing for any length of time with both feet flat on the floor. Whenever possible, get one foot up onto a step or a stool. Of course, you will find yourself in situations where this kind of relief is not to be found, such as at a cocktail party where all the chairs have been moved out, and everybody has to stand around, flatfooted.

Department-store shopping can be painful, too. Most stores provide little seating and no foot rails. But there is usually some solution if you look hard enough. For example, if you take the escalators, not the elevator, you can stand on one step and rest one foot on the step above.

I was going to suggest supermarkets as a bad place, too, but at least you can rest one foot on the lower shelf of your shopping cart.

That's right. And while you're pushing the cart, you can lean over and take some of your upper body weight on your arms. As I mentioned earlier, varying your posture usually gives your back some relief.

Art galleries are difficult places for back sufferers. Typically they offer no place to sit down and nothing but miles of level floor, except for a staircase here and there. Most other indoor exhibitions and fairs can be just as difficult.

Now that you mention it, I realize that's probably why my back hurts whenever I have to stand around a long time waiting for a bus. Maybe I should try using the curb as a foot-rest.

That's not a bad idea if there's no danger from the traffic. Standing with one foot on your lunch box or briefcase is one good strategy. Even leaning against a building or a lamp-post will often help a little.

Yes. I've already discovered that, especially if I'm carrying a heavy package I don't want to put down. Are there any rules about carrying heavy objects?

Yes. I often tell my patients, "Never take out the garbage in your Sunday suit."

You've got to be kidding. If I have to carry out the garbage, what difference does it make whether I'm wearing good clothes or old ones?

I'm serious. If you're wearing your good clean clothes, you will instinctively hold the garbage bag away from your body. When you reach out and hold a load at arm's length, there's a leverage effect. The distance between your spine and the load magnifies the strain on your back. If that garbage is heavy, you can easily bring on a bout of back pain.

The most basic principle of all, when it comes to lifting any object, is to bring it in close to your body – hug it if you can – and save your back that way. This one fact is more important than all the other instructions you've heard about lifting with your back straight or bending your knees. If I thought people would take the idea seriously, I'd distribute a bumper-sticker asking, HAVE YOU HUGGED YOUR GARBAGE CAN TODAY?

Do you find more back problems among people who have to do a lot of standing, compared to people who are seated during much of a normal day?

It may not seem logical but sitting down is harder on the back than standing up. Sitting places a greater load on the discs in your spine. And that prolonged compression may cause changes in a disc, flattening it out somewhat and squeezing the material inside towards the outer shell. That sort of pressure can be painful.

Then I suppose it is a big help to sit in a comfortable chair.

The kind of seat you use can make a tremendous difference, but I would be careful with the word "comfortable." One of the great horrors in the world of chairdom is the so-called "comfy" chair – that overstuffed monster that looks inviting but feels almost as if it were designed to produce backache. Its arms are so high that you can't rest your own arms on them. The seat is so deep from front to back that you can't rest your feet comfortably on the floor. And the back of the chair is so soft that it provides no support. Your spine sags so much as you slump into it that you are forced into a flexed position. And the more "give" there is to the back of the chair, the more you have to bend forward to compensate.

A "comfy" chair looks comfortable because it is soft. Nobody likes the idea of sitting on a hard chair. But you have to sit in a "comfy" chair for only a short time to realize it is actually a back-trap.

Then am I better off with the other extreme – say, a hard bench?

Not necessarily. The hard, backless bench – the kind you see in many shopping-malls – can be almost as bad. But at least it allows you a choice of posture. If you find yourself having to use a bench like that, try sitting the way football players often do: hunched forward, with your hands or elbows on your knees. Taking the weight through your arms unloads your spine. In fact it's a great position for a three-minute rest, but if you stay that way too long you'll find that when you straighten up your back feels sore. Maybe that's what shopping-mall designers intend – making sure you won't sit too long without getting up and going into a store to buy something.

A bench, unlike the "comfy" chair, allows you to choose your own position and lets you change that position as often as you choose. I can think of eight or ten ways I might sit on an ordinary backless bench, and each one would provide some relief by varying the otherwise constant load on my spine. Even so, without a firm back support and suitable arm-rests, the bench is far from ideal.

Another difficult form of a seat is the Cape Cod chair, a wooden outdoor lounging chair with a seat quite close to the ground. The Cape Code has wide, flat arms and a back that tilts twenty degrees or so away from the vertical. The seat has wooden slats that slope sharply downward from front to back. It looks comfortably inviting, but, as you discover once you're seated, it's very awkward to get up again.

Most backache sufferers have had bad experiences as well with director's chairs, which have curved canvas backs that provide no support for the spine, and narrow seats that make position changes difficult.

Sometimes I wonder if there isn't a world-wide chair conspiracy against people with back problems, especially when I see modern chairs made of chrome or stainless steel that are so uncomfortable for the spine. Even the bean-bag chair, which has the merit of adapting itself comfortably to your body shape, can be as hard to get out of as the Cape Cod.

Is there such a thing as the perfect chair?

No, there isn't. We are not all the same shape and size, and the chair that suits one person may not suit another. A colleague of mine, a plastic surgeon, now retired, didn't like performing surgery while sitting on a standard stool. Instead he had his own seat designed. It looked for all the world like a big, old-fashioned tractor seat. To him, it was the ultimate in working comfort. And he wasn't alone. Whenever he was out of the operating room, several other surgeons used to compete for the privilege of sitting in that seat. But not everybody found it comfortable.

Of course you stand a better chance of achieving near perfection if you know exactly what you want and can afford to have it custom made.

I once visited the shop of a craftsman who specializes in custom-making chairs for maximum comfort. He had a simple system using a heavy mesh screen and movable wooden rods to shape a chair exactly to the contours of your back – and your backside. I was quite taken with his approach; he didn't try to impress me with a lot of scientific theory about the biomechanics of my spine. He just worked hard to make absolutely sure the end result would suit me perfectly. His whole approach was: "Let's build whatever feels comfortable to you."

What guidelines can you offer to a person who is looking for a good chair for an office job?

Find a chair that supports the small of your back with its normal forward curve, without rigidity or too much "give." The back of the chair should tilt backwards ten to twenty degrees, to suit your comfort and needs, and it should have a means of being locked into place at the angle you prefer. Make sure the seat is deep enough to support the length of your thighs and wide enough to allow easy position change. If you're going to be seated for long periods, you want to be able to shift from one side to another, to cross and uncross your legs, lean forward, lean back, and so on, to ease the stress.

The chair you're looking for should have arm-rests that allow you to transfer some weight from the upper body and temporarily reduce the load on your lower spine.

Check the height of the chair seat against your desk or work table to ensure that they combine to place your work surface at the level of your elbows when you are seated with your arms at your sides and your forearms held parallel to the floor. The chair should also let you rest your feet easily on the floor, to reduce the amount of weight taken by the backs of your thighs.

And even with the best possible chair, you might do well to place a stool or even a thick book on the floor in front of you, so you can prop one foot up now and then. Or do what I do: pull out a low desk drawer and rest your foot on that.

Is it a good idea to have a seat that can be easily raised and lowered?

With an adjustable chair, a person can obtain the seating height that seems exactly right, although this can also be achieved by trying out various chairs of fixed height. It seems like a good idea to vary the height of your seating from time to time while you work, but in my experience few people use adjustable chairs this way.

What about that new "kneeling chair," which has a seat with an extreme forward slope and a knee-rest that places nearly all your body weight on your knees. Does it employ some useful scientific principle?

The kneeling position automatically puts the forward curve of the low back into a neutral position, and that's good. But the design also puts a substantial load on your knees, and some older people may not like that for long. I wouldn't buy this chair just on the basis of how it feels during a tryout in the store; I'd want to test it personally during several days of actual use. Over time, you might find it very comfortable or you might discover that the kneeling chair is too confining since it deprives you of the chance to change position easily. Like many devices built to help the back, it's great for some and not so good for others.

Is there such a thing as the perfect way to sit?

The best position, for your back's sake, is probably a compromise between sitting rigidly upright, in the old schoolroom tradition, and slumping way down, as teenagers often do when watching TV or talking on the phone.

A couple of guidelines, based on biomechanics, are worth keeping in mind. First, forward bending increases disc load. So don't bend forward for long periods. Second, try to find some support for your lower back, from the chair itself, from a small cushion, or from a specially designed support.

Aren't specially designed supports just commercial gimmicks?

No, I consider them legitimate because they induce a posture that is physiologically normal – a forward curve at the neck, a backward curve of the thoracic spine, in the area of the shoulders, and a forward curve in the lumbar region, or lower spine. If you can maintain those curves in their correct proportions, you will go far in relieving your back pain. Of course, the advantages of an expensive contour support must be weighed against the benefits of a simple, inexpensive cushion. The choice depends on comfort, convenience, and cost.

So proper sitting posture means avoiding extreme positions?

Most of the time, yes. But even the extremes – slumping down and sitting bolt upright – can be used as brief variations to provide helpful relief. We all know that if we stay in any one position for long, such as in a movie theater or on a long car ride, our bodies and legs become cramped and sore. Sometimes a change is as good as a rest.

But what if you have to work at a desk with a knee hole so narrow and low that there's no room to use a foot-rest or cross your legs or move around much?

Try shifting occasionally from side to side, riding "side saddle," so to speak. Also, stand up and walk around two or three times an hour, to loosen up your muscles and joints.

So, that's another regular strategy to use – loosening up by moving around now and then.

That's right, and if you're on the lookout for chances to limber up, you'll sometimes find them in surprising places. For example, at Toronto's Pearson Airport, Terminal One contains several staircases that seem quite inconvenient to arriving passengers.

As you make your way to the luggage carousel, you have to walk down narrow flights of stairs and then cope with a door that will not stay open by itself. It's awkward, especially for anyone toting carry-on baggage, but it has one big advantage: it provides useful exercise for passengers who may have been sitting in a plane for several hours with their backs and legs fairly immobile. Getting down that staircase and opening that door involve walking, flexing, twisting, and pushing with the arms. All these motions help you stretch, and they may be especially welcome if you have common backache.

This short interlude of exercise can be helpful even if you have used all my standard tricks to protect your spine during the flight – sitting with one foot up on a small case, keeping the seat belt tightly fastened, supporting the hollow in the low back with a small pillow, and choosing an aisle seat so you can get up easily and move about.

How would you rate the average airplane seat compared to the typical automobile seat?

For most people the airplane seat is a little better, but it's always a matter of personal preference. Some new car seat designs are very good but even the best of them will give some people back-aches. One good step in car design would be to do away with the bench seat. Among the horror tales of bad seating, the familiar bench ranks right up there with the "comfy" chair.

Several years ago, I had a car I couldn't drive without a seat cushion. I got a nasty backache whenever I sat in the driver's seat without a pillow wedged behind the small of my back. If my children didn't want me going out, they'd hide my pillow. When I bought another car, I assumed I'd need the pillow, as always. But in the new car I found the pillow quite uncomfortable, and I discarded it. I've found it's wrong to make any absolute rule about your back and its needs, since they will vary from one situation to another.

Later I got a car with a steering wheel that tilts and a power seat that's adjustable every which way. Now I'd hate to be without those extras. Driving on a long trip you can assume many different positions. You can ride for a while like a bus driver, with the seat high and the steering wheel up close and almost horizontal, like a sundial. Or you can place the steering wheel almost vertical, like a clock on a wall, and then sit back as though driving a sports car. And between those two extremes there are a dozen possible variations.

What about other types of vehicles – bicycles, for instance? Are they hard on the back?

The biggest drawback to the bicycle is the small size of the seat. With a racing bike, especially, a large proportion of your body weight bears down on a relatively small surface, and so the concentration of load is high. This effect is somewhat offset by the fact that you are carrying much of your upper body weight on your arms. But that forward-bent position creates more load on the discs, so some of that advantage is nullified. If you have back problems, choose a conventional bicycle, not a racer.

I suppose motorcycle seats are pretty bad for backs.

Not necessarily. The motorcycle seat has evolved from a bicycle-style seat into a small bench, usually with a big pommel, and that's an improvement. Some motorcycles also have arm- and back-rests, which of course take some of the load off the spine.

What about horseback riding – is that bad for your back?

Not really. A good rider adopts a posture that is upright without being stiffly military, and that's good.

But what about the jarring effect when a horse trots or canters?

For beginners, that's a hazard, but once people learn to ride properly, they reduce that impact with their legs, minimizing the shock to their spines. Of course, most of us will have some backache after a long day in the saddle.

Earlier, you mentioned a colleague who liked to work on a tractor-type seat. Isn't it ironical that your back is better off when you drive a tractor than when you sit behind the wheel of a luxury automobile?

It's better off only because of the wide, contour seat that used to be standard on every tractor. Unfortunately, modern tractors have cabs with bench seats, which are hard on the back. The driver's back is subjected to a lot of jarring as he drives over rough terrain, but the worst punishment for his spine may come from vibration. Studies have shown that certain rates of vibration produce a corresponding resonance in the spine. If a machine vibrates at a certain frequency, and if that frequency happens to match the natural resonance of the spine, it will create waves of movement that can seriously aggravate back trouble.

This phenomenon explains why many people who do certain kinds of work – operating earth-movers, for instance – suffer from backache. It applies also to some truck drivers and, in fact, to almost any job where the person's body is subjected to constant vibration.

Is backache inevitable, then, for people in jobs like those?

I wouldn't say it's inevitable, but it's much more likely. Some people can go through a lot of physical aggravation without developing chronic backache. But even the people who are vulnerable can take steps to ward off trouble. Much of the vibration can be reduced, if not eliminated, by the use of spring-mounted seats or padding, or by better design of the machinery itself. There is a lot of research going on now to find out what vibrations are harmful and how they can be reduced, changed, or eliminated.

Does vibration cause a particular condition that you can diagnose?

No, vibration just accentuates the same kind of wear in the discs and back joints that you'd find in any patient with common backache.

You said earlier that sitting is harder on the back than standing. Are you better off, then, with a job where you sit for maybe an hour or two and then get up and do some other form of work?

It depends. That kind of job is great if you get up to move around, stretch, or do light work. It's not so good if you have to go from being sedentary to suddenly doing heavy lifting. This happens, for instance, with a truck driver who does his own loading and unloading. He works hard loading his truck for an hour or two, then drives for several hours while his back and legs stiffen up, and then jumps out of his cab and begins hoisting heavy objects again. It's hardly surprising when pain results from that abuse of a spine already affected by the normal wear and tear of aging.

But if that's his job, he can hardly avoid the problem.

Maybe not entirely, but he would be smart to take a tip from professional athletes, who know the importance of warming up before any strenuous activity. Before he tackles a loading job, the driver should walk briskly around his rig and do a little bending and stretching, maybe on the pretext of checking his tires or examining the freight. Anything to prepare the back muscles for the exertion ahead.

What other occupations are particularly difficult for people with back problems?

It's hard to think of a job that doesn't have some potential for causing backache, although some jobs, of course, are worse than others. Construction workers and dock hands often get backaches because they do a lot of bending, lifting, and twisting of the upper body. Nurses are vulnerable, too, often having to lift bedridden patients. The trouble usually starts with the unexpected lift or twist. The person has just started to lift when his partner drops the other end of a heavy box, or he accidentally slips on a wet floor and twists hard to avoid falling down. In such cases, the sudden load catches the muscles by surprise and the spine has to take most of the weight.

One of the toughest jobs on the back is hard-rock mining. To drill holes where dynamite sticks will be inserted into the rock face, a man has to lift a hundred-pound power hammer and hold it at shoulder height while it vibrates like mad. If any job can be described as back-breaking work, that's it. There are machines that can help do the job, but much of hard-rock mining is still done with human muscle – and backs. Hard-rock miners are a strong breed, and they need all that strength to protect their spines. For instance, if they have weak belly muscles, the load on their backs may just be too much.

A jack-hammer operator working on a paved street is a little better off, not having to bear the whole weight of the equipment while using it. But he must lift that heavy hammer continually, often twisting his upper body as he does so. His back would be a lot better off if he used his feet to turn his whole body at once.

Some other occupations belong on this "high risk" list, such as repetitious assembly-line jobs requiring lifting and turning from fixed positions. To increase my understanding of these causes of backache, I've toured many factories, including one where fire hoses are manufactured. There, workers use long metal poles to handle masses of rubbery goo, which they lift at arm's length and mix with a twisting motion. If any of them avoid chronic backache, I'd like to know how.

Some sheet-metal workers have to lift heavy materials and tools in positions that strain their backs. House painters are asking for trouble if they stand on ladders and reach out awkwardly with their scrapers and paint brushes. Proper scaffolding, as well as being safer, provides much more comfort for the back.

And speaking of ladders, I mustn't forget to mention firefighting. It's hard to think of a greater challenge to a person's back than climbing up and down a ladder under the most urgent and stressful conditions while toting a heavy fire hose or carrying a fire victim to safety. Firefighters often have to lift other heavy objects as well. One fireman told me how he once had to reach out at arm's length and turn over a rowboat, single-handed, to get at a fire he was fighting.

Even the man who drives the fire engine lets himself in for back problems. He has to manage a huge steering wheel and operate a heavy clutch while bouncing along at high speed.

Flying a helicopter is even harder on the back than driving a fire engine. In flight, the pilot has both feet elevated to operate the rudder pedals, a posture that puts extra stress on the discs. He must keep both arms in action, with engine vibration constantly jarring his spine. One of my patients is a firefighter who moonlights as a helicopter flight instructor. I can't think of a worse combination.

It's a real tribute to the strength of the human system that, although so many jobs produce a high incidence of backache, there is little real damage done to the spine. And vigorous physical conditioning of the muscles of the back and belly can substantially reduce the discomfort.

What about outdoor chores?

Many people develop sore backs doing yard jobs, especially jobs they do only occasionally. Snow shoveling is a prime example. Being seasonal, it's not routine. It involves a lot of lifting, twisting, and turning, all done under cold conditions. And, typically, a householder intent on clearing a sidewalk or driveway won't take the time to warm up to the task. It's an open invitation to back trouble. Powered snow-blowers may be hazardous for other reasons but they're a boon to back pain sufferers.

Can you suggest a specific strategy for people who shovel snow by hand?

Yes – first, dress warmly, particularly over the back. Cold air can tighten the back muscles. If you're about to do a lot of heavy work, run through a short warm-up routine before you go outside. When you shovel snow, lift light loads. Remember: you don't have to clear the whole sidewalk in one shovelful. Carry the snow where you want it, rather than trying to fling it a great distance. And if you're throwing the snow to one side, turn your feet as you do so – don't twist your spine. The job may take a little longer that way, but you'll save yourself a lot of pain.

Some of the same principles apply to grass cutting. Avoid extreme positions, such as bending forward excessively. Work in stages. If your back is sore and the job is likely to take two hours of steady work, spread the task over four or five hours, resting or doing entirely different kinds of jobs in between.

Hedge trimming can be hard on the back, because you often have to hold the clippers at arm's length. Power clippers get the job done faster, of course, but they're also heavier, causing extra strain.

Raking grass or leaves can be another problem. To avoid un-necessary bending or reaching, rake with short strokes, using your arms and shoulders, or moving forward or backward with your legs. Keep your spine fairly erect and as relaxed as possible.

If you are hauling firewood, don't carry an uncomfortably large load. And give the task some variety. For example, you might carry the wood in a relay pattern: first, several trips in from the woodpile to the bottom of the porch steps; then a second sequence, up the steps and into the house. That way, the job becomes less of an endurance test. In many yard jobs, some strain may be unavoidable, but you can reduce it by resting intermittently, if only for a minute or two each time.

I remind you, though, that these chores won't actually harm your back; they'll just make it sore. Going at any task the wrong way may make life unpleasant for you, but it won't actually damage your spine. It can put up with a lot of abuse; you just don't want to push things to the point where it can't take any more without protesting painfully.

Think of it as a sort of bank account: every time you place some strain on your back, you're drawing on its reserves. Every time you rest or perform muscle-strengthening exercises, you're making a "deposit," restoring some resilience to your "back account." That's why it is so important to take those intermittent rest periods between stressful tasks.

What about the indoor chores that most homemakers perform? Can you suggest special strategies for them?

You can easily strain your spine quite unnecessarily doing many ordinary household tasks – vacuuming a carpet, ironing clothes, making beds, lifting objects from high shelves. The most important principle is to find the most comfortable – or, as the case may be, the least awkward – way of doing the job.

If you're running a vacuum cleaner, keep your back in a comfortable position and move your arms and legs. Lunge forward with your legs and reach with your arms while holding your back erect. See yourself demonstrating the grace of a fencing master.

If you're bending over to make a bed, try to bend at the hips and keep your back relaxed or even slightly arched like a ballet dancer's. Or use a knee bend if that's practical. Some people even kneel on the floor while tucking the blankets and sheets under the mattress.

Instead of straining to lift an object from a shelf at arm's length, use a step stool to get close. Remember, that's the most important principle to observe during any kind of lifting or carrying: hold the object as close to your body as you can and keep it there.

At the ironing board, stand with one foot up, on a low box, for instance. If your back is really sore, try ironing sitting down on a stool or a high chair. Change positions frequently. Sit on a stool or even a countertop while you're waiting for that kettle to boil. Move often and give your back a rest once in a while by leaning on your arms to take the weight of your upper body. Standing over the sink is easier when you put one foot on a shelf inside a cupboard.

Any special advice about moving furniture?

The best strategy of all is to use devices, rather than muscle power, whenever you can – a handcart is better than a back for toting a refrigerator, for instance. And with a little ingenuity, you can often improvise. To move a heavy appliance across a smooth floor, for example, you can often tip it onto a thick blanket and then drag it quite easily. If you must use your own power, let your legs or arms help your spine handle the strain.

It sounds to me as though most people face the risk of backache whether they're at home or out on the job. What are the main points to remember if they want to avoid it?

One very important thing is to keep your muscles, especially your stomach muscles, in good shape, through good postural habits and proper exercise.

Look for ways to modify your regular tasks to reduce the strain or risk. Or, in the case of sedentary jobs, find ways to provide variations in your sitting or standing position. Some people who must stand at a counter all day, for instance, might sit occasionally on a high stool.

If you work at a desk or counter, take note that the comfortable height for the work surface is about level with your elbows. Since the same height can't suit everybody, some enlightened employers now provide platforms, adjustable chairs, or varied or adjustable work surfaces, to keep everyone comfortable.

If possible, give your back short rest breaks several times through-out the day.

And, of course, use the back-saving techniques I've described for bending, lifting, handling tools and materials, and so on.

Could you say a little more about lifting? I'm surprised you haven't emphasized that if you have to lift a heavy object off the ground, you should crouch down and do the lifting with your legs, rather than bending over and straining your back.

Well, that's the time-honored advice. But some current evidence suggests that it may not matter whether you lift mainly with your legs or actually bend over and use your back instead. The important thing, as I said earlier, is to "hug" the load so as to avoid lifting it at arm's length. The key is the distance between the load and the spine. The shorter the distance, the shorter the lever arm, in engineering terms, and the smaller the force required in the back muscles to offset the load. And of course that means a lot less pressure on the spine.

Using your legs to lift is fine in most circumstances, but it isn't always possible. You can't do that for instance if you are hauling an outboard motor out of the trunk of a car. Or if you are lifting a large box, you may not be able to squat down and still get your arms around it. Also, if you're especially tired, you're not likely to use the "leg lift" method, because it requires a great deal more energy than just using your back. The body always seems to prefer the most economical way of doing any job.

So, you see, there is no single correct way to lift; it depends on the situation. Try to use your legs and shoulder muscles when you can, let gravity and the object's momentum work for you, and don't forget to hug.

A second important principle for safe lifting is to avoid the twisting action of the upper body I mentioned earlier. Discs don't like to be twisted. If you must turn while lifting, turn with your feet, not with your trunk.

Many people know how to lift properly but ignore what they know. They should keep reminding themselves of what's best for their backs. But let me say it once again: even if you hurt your back while lifting a few more pounds of load than you can handle, you almost never damage it. But for most of us, "hurt" – even though it's not the same as "harm" – is more trouble than we need. Especially if our backs remain sore enough to interfere with daily living for several days.

Would you go so far as to say that some people whose backs bother them on the job should try to find some other line of work?

That's a good suggestion in theory, but it's not that easy these days to find a new job, let alone an alternative type of work.

I feel sorry for people who inadvertently get into jobs their backs simply can't handle, and I feel even sorrier for those who develop back pain after years in one job and can find no way of switching to other work. One of my patients is a middle-aged police officer who had major surgery for spinal stenosis, a condition I will talk about later. After the operation his back was much better but not normal, by any means. His superiors wanted him to get right back into harness, as a uniformed patrol officer, but he dreaded the prospect of having to spend each shift in a cruiser. On patrol, he has to sit for hours at a time on a badly sprung car seat, with the weight of a holster, gun belt, and gun all pulling on his back muscles. In the winter, his back bears the extra weight of a heavy coat. And there is always the chance that apprehending a suspect might require heavy physical exertion.

Well, he went back to work, and for the first few weeks managed to get posted to courtroom duty. But, the last I heard, he was under pressure to return to his regular assignment. He told me that if he resisted much longer, he'd likely be fired. If he went back and couldn't cope, he'd probably be fired anyway.

Another patient of mine had a different problem. He's a radiologist specializing in angiography, the X-ray study of blood vessels. Routinely, he puts on a lead apron that weighs about twelve pounds (5.5 kg) and bends over the X-ray table to inject contrast material into patients' arteries. Because of his backache, he couldn't do that work for more than a few minutes at a time. When I saw him he was already on disability leave and was considering changing his specialty to something less demanding. But that meant throwing away twelve years' experience to start training for something new.

Those are just a couple of examples of occupational problems for which there are no easy solutions.

I can see where a lead apron would cause trouble, but what about some of the commoner items people wear? For instance, I've heard that women shouldn't wear high-heeled shoes. Do you advise your patients to give them up?

No. I consider that unrealistic and somewhat unnecessary. High heels may increase the curve in the small of the back (doctors call it the lumbar lordosis), and this posture can lead to backache. But high heels don't harm the spine – nor, incidentally, do low heels automatically make a woman's back feel better.

If high heels are causing a problem, I suggest several simple strategies that many women already use as a matter of course. Avoid standing for long periods. Or take along a second, more comfortable, pair of shoes and use them intermittently. Or, in a casual situation, walk around in stocking feet.

What do you advise back patients to do when choosing a pair of shoes?

New shoes should feel comfortable almost from the moment you put them on. I tell my patients, "You're not breaking in the shoes; you're breaking down your feet." The height of the heel affects the posture of the spine. The width of the shoe determines the pressure on the toes. When you stand up, your foot widens under the weight of your body, and that's when the fit of the shoe can be determined most accurately.

What about jogging shoes?

My first inclination is to advise back patients not to take up jogging at all. But if jogging is your choice as a recreational sport, I suggest you get jogging shoes that are well-cushioned, to soften the impact on the spine. The heels should be broad to minimize the natural torque action of running – that is, the slight rotation of the leg at the knee.

Could you explain more about "torque action"? If rotation is natural, as you said, why should joggers need shoes with broad heels to prevent it?

If you'd spent your life running all day every day, your knees would develop a tolerance for that increased rotation. But most joggers aren't seasoned runners, and it's easy for them to push their bodies beyond their normal experience.

What is your main objection to jogging?

I don't necessarily object to jogging, although I do feel the joggers I see should be given only one of two choices: they can jog or they can complain. The most important factors are the total mileage (distances under two miles a day generally don't cause trouble) and the running surface. I see nothing wrong with jogging on grass, cinders, or a sprung track. But people are just asking for trouble by jogging on concrete or asphalt – their feet, knees, and backs can't take that kind of punishment.

If you want to give your heart and lungs a regular workout, you can choose one of several exercises that are just as effective as jogging, with less potential for back pain. These include swimming, certain aerobic exercises without a great deal of bouncing up and down, and fast walking – not Olympic-speed walking, just walking briskly. Walking doesn't have the glamour of running, but it's an excellent cardiovascular exercise.

Are there a lot of other recreational sports that may cause wear and tear on your spine?

Most athletic activities don't cause wear and tear; they just aggravate what you have already developed naturally. Every activity causes *some* strain on your back, and your spine has no trouble keeping it under control. The unfortunate cases occur when people go to extremes and actually cause heavy wear on their spines quite needlessly. One patient of mine was a well-built man in his twenties who came to me complaining of severe back pain. And no wonder. He was working out regularly with bar-bells, using routines he had invented, without any understanding of what their effects might be.

For instance, he would take a fifteen-pound (7 kg) weight in each hand, extend his arms at shoulder height, and then swing his whole upper torso back and forth as hard as he could, in violent rotations that must have had his discs pleading for mercy. And he was routinely doing a thousand repetitions every day.

I explained to him that while a healthy back can put up with almost anything, discs hate violent twisting. He'd been asking for trouble – and he got it. His objective had been to keep his mid-section fit and trim. But, as I told him, there are many exercises that will do that without placing all the strain on the discs. Side bends will usually keep anyone's middle-age spread under control. Slow, resisted rotations on an exercise machine can strengthen the waist muscles that protect the discs, and can do so without injuring the spine in the process. Even running or walking can do a lot to tighten the waistline.

I'm not suggesting that this young man's back was ruined for life, but he was inflicting a lot of needless wear and tear for a result that could be achieved in several painless ways.

Is pain a pretty accurate indication that a particular sport is bad for your back?

Not at all. As long as your common sense keeps you from going to extremes, you can consider playing almost any sport you enjoy. If you're a 150-pound, forty-five-year-old male with a disc problem, you will obviously decline to get out onto a field to play serious football against a lineup of 300-pounders. But it's a mistake, in my view, to avoid a friendly game of basketball, or an afternoon of tennis, just because you know your back will start hurting. It's a tradeoff: if you like the activity, that pain is the price you pay for the recreational and social enjoyment you get from the game.

I have a booklet published by a drug company for doctors to hand out to their back patients. It is filled with all sorts of silly advice, the silliest of which is a list of "good" and "bad" exercises. Never mind the fact that what's "bad" for one back patient might be perfectly okay for another, this company plays the whole thing so safe it's laughable. What happened, I'm sure, was that their lawyer said, "Look, we can't afford to have our name on this booklet if there is even the slightest possibility of somebody getting hurt after taking our advice."

The result was that virtually every popular sport appears on the "bad" list: tennis, golf, squash, basketball, volleyball – you name it. The "good" sports column is limited to such innocuous activities as swimming and slow walking. I wondered why they didn't include tiddly-winks, window-shopping, and indoor bird-watching.

The underlying message is that people with back problems aren't allowed to have any fun – which is sheer nonsense.

Do you have your own list of sports that are good or bad for people with back problems?

No, I don't think of them that way. Some sports entail risks even for people with healthy backs – hang-gliding, ski-jumping, sky-diving, boxing, wrestling – not just because they impose a strain on your spine but because they entail the risk of serious injury to other parts of the body, which is a completely different thing.

We have to assume for the purpose of this discussion that you will be careful enough and lucky enough not to get seriously injured in the sport of your choice. With that proviso, I see no need for a list of "safe" and "unsafe" sports. Virtually every sport involves some strain on your back, and virtually every back can stand it.

Then how can I make the choice from among the sports that appeal to me?

It helps to understand that strain on your back may take three distinct forms: placing extra weight on your spinal discs, arching your spine and loading the small joints, and rotating your trunk to produce that twisting effect I described.

Once you're aware of these causes of strain, you don't need medical training to decide which of them are involved in the sport of your choice and whether the satisfaction and fun will be worth the resulting discomfort or pain. Barring accidents, you won't actually harm your back engaging in the popular sports you might choose, and it's ridiculous to avoid any activity just because it may hurt a little at the time or produce some stiffness or soreness the next day.

What sort of activity places extra weight on your spine?

Extra weight can mean either literally taking on an extra burden, as you do in weight-lifting, or producing a pounding action on the discs, for instance by running on a hard surface. Sports that load extra weight on your spine include curling, bowling, horseback riding, dirt biking, hunting, and fishing.

Once you understand the basic mechanics, you can easily figure out how to reduce the hazard, by adopting certain techniques or simply by going at it less vigorously. If you haven't bowled for several weeks, restrict yourself to just a game or two, with intervals of rest. If you go fishing, be careful how you lift that outboard motor from the car trunk, and don't try to manhandle that big canoe ashore all by yourself. When you are hunting in the bush, keep your pack light and let someone else carry out the moose. On horseback or a dirt bike, choose the trail carefully and save your back by making your legs absorb those bounces and jolts.

What are the sports that force you to arch your back?

You arch your back at some time in nearly every popular recreational sport: basketball, tennis, badminton, volleyball, hockey, baseball, skiing, and certain styles of swimming, notably the breaststroke. Arching the back is inherent in the actions of rowing, canoeing, and archery.

Is there anything I can do, then, if I'm determined to play one of those "arching" sports and it makes my back hurt?

If your problem is in the small joints of your spine, arching your back may cause pain. It's impossible to avoid that posture completely, but you can avoid extreme positions by practicing a pelvic tilt to flatten your lower back a little; I'll describe the pelvic tilt in more detail later when we talk about exercises. Rest during the game by bending forward slightly – and resolve to live with the remaining discomfort as part of a fair tradeoff.

I can see where many of the "arching" sports also involve twisting or rotating the upper part of your body.

That's true. Baseball and tennis are two examples. But the worst offenders are squash, racketball, and golf. Compared to those racket sports, golf may seem pretty sedate, but, in fact, a well-executed golf swing places an enormous rotational strain on your spine. Even so, if you play golf you can learn to modify your swing to reduce the strain. Using an exercise machine to practice careful, resisted rotations can strengthen the trunk muscles and help protect the discs from sudden, twisting movements. And, with any sport, you can practice moderation in one way or another, playing less intensely or for shorter periods and taking longer or more frequent rests.

About the "tradeoff" you mentioned – is it just for professionals and ambitious amateurs, or should ordinary people go on playing sports in spite of back pain?

Anybody can make a tradeoff – and many ordinary people do, simply because the enjoyment and satisfaction outweigh the pain. Two of my male patients are among the most enthusiastic jocks I've ever met, but they are not exceptional athletes, just ordinary people who enjoy exercise and friendly competition. One is a forty-nine-year-old with disc trouble. He loves to play hockey. Sometimes, during a tournament, he'll play two or three games in one week. Often, his back pain begins just as he bends forward to lace up his skates, and sometimes it gets so bad he has to leave the game. But he keeps going back for more.

The other fellow, also middle-aged, is an avid windsurfer. I can't think of a sport where the back is arched more acutely; and the weight-loading factor is considerable, too. This man has some problems with wear in his spinal joints that may need surgical attention some day. But you would have to lock him up to keep him off that sailboard.

Both men put up with a fair amount of pain and stiffness in order to participate in the sports they enjoy so much. I can't think of a better tradeoff than that – and, obviously, neither can they.

Could they actually help their backs that way, in the long run, by staying active?

Only in the general sense that they are building up muscular strength that may help protect their spines from unnecessary strain. But, like most competitive or recreational sports, hockey and windsurfing are far from being remedies for back pain. What these two men *are* doing is refusing to let back pain keep them on the sidelines. Both men also make a regular habit of doing specific exercises to strengthen their backs – an entirely different matter, which we will discuss in the final chapter.

The important thing to point out here is that whatever activity you may engage in – from toting a garbage bag to climbing a mountain peak – you can use techniques that will minimize the effects of natural aging on your spine. It's up to you to decide whether a particular activity is worth the stiffness or pain it will produce.

It's also up to you to adopt or devise strategies and make personal choices to ensure that you, not your spine, will determine the quality and style of the life you lead.

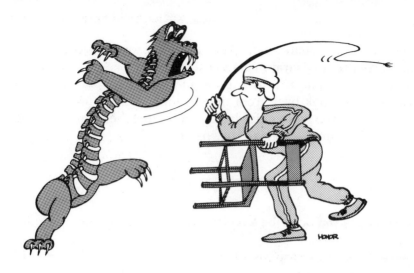

2. *TAMING THE BEAST*

There is no denying the fact that virtually everyone with a back problem will experience painful episodes from time to time.

I often tell my patients once they're pain free, it would be to their benefit if they could have one more acute episode which they could successfully abort. That way, they would discover for themselves that they are in control. This observation is based on my experience with thousands of patients who have trained themselves to ward off an attack and then actually done so. If they have faced and tamed the beast even once, they no longer have reason to fear it.

One of the great satisfactions of my work is to have a patient come in and say, "I just had a bad attack last week, but I knew what to do, and now I'm fine."

Even before you reach that stage, however, there is one consolation to keep in mind: *without exception, every acute attack eventually subsides.* It may be hard to remember at the time – and even harder to believe – but no pain attack, no matter how severe, will stay with you indefinitely. It will always get better.

What you can usefully remember, too, is that as long as you are taking the right steps to look after your back, no attack will return you to square one. There is always some residue of gain from your previous training and exercise.

As long as you are making the proper effort, you will find it satisfying to look back from time to time, to see how far you've come. And even more satisfying to realize that the beast is, indeed, thoroughly tamed – and you are in control.

How would you describe a typical attack of back pain?

As with so many aspects of back pain, people's problems with acute attacks vary from one individual to another. Pain is the common feature, but it is not the same type or intensity for everyone, and it is certainly not constant.

One of the stories I often hear from people who have had minor attacks is that they are immobilized by the terrible fear that "something is going wrong" with their backs. I know the feeling. When it comes over me, I know instinctively that if I try to move I am going to trigger some pain. For all practical purposes, I feel trapped in one position.

In other words, you are paralyzed by your back pain?

Not actually. Paralysis is a very exact term denoting the loss of muscle power due to a disruption of the normal nerve impulses. What we're talking about here is a powerful psychological inhibition against movement. Your body "knows" that movement will cause pain and refuses to let you try it.

The trick, then, is to assume and remain in the most soothing rest position you can find. There is no single correct position. I remember one patient who was comfortable only on his hands and knees, and he even stayed in bed that way. You should experiment gently until you find a position that works for you. Most rest positions remove the loading effect of gravity and restore the neutral curve of the spine. If you are able to do that, you can, in most cases, eliminate the pain almost completely.

I think some people who have had severe attacks will find that hard to believe.

I'm sure they will. My comments apply to typical attacks, but the amount and character of the pain can range across a wide spectrum. At one extreme, the pain is immediate and so severe that the person may actually fall to the floor. The severity depends on several factors, including the source of the pain, the degree of muscle spasm, and the amount of fear.

But even in the worst attacks, the pain is typically intermittent. If a patient describes back pain as constant – twenty-four hours a day without change – and if the physical examination shows evidence of nothing but natural wear and tear, I can be sure the pain is being aggravated by the person's emotional responses.

What's the first thing a person should know about coping with an acute attack?

Timing is critical. The sooner you can take action the better, because the longer the muscles remain cramped, the more they become irritated and likely to continue in spasm. In time, they begin to retain fluid. And that extra fluid – medically it's called edema – swells the muscles, increases the muscles' irritability, and creates more pain.

Are you saying that back pain is simply a spasm of the back muscles?

Not precisely. But usually the most important pain-producing factor in an acute attack is the accompanying muscle spasm. You want to help the muscle relax as quickly as possible. Sometimes all it takes is a little bit of positioning and gentle stretching, much like getting out of bed to walk off that cramp you get in the calf of your leg. Sometimes aborting the acute attack can be as simple as sitting down and hugging your knees to your chest. Or sometimes squatting can provide the relief you need.

Or you could try doing what I sometimes do. When I have an attack, I lie on the floor with my feet and calves resting on the seat of a chair and my body close underneath, so that my knees are right above my chest. If you had a side view of me in that position, I'd look like the letter "Z." Then I place a thin cushion under my buttocks, to raise my hips slightly. This position takes the tension out of my back.

But in some settings, don't you feel pretty foolish suddenly getting down and lying on the floor like that?

Of course I do, so I try to get away where I'm not the center of attention. But it's a tradeoff: better that than looking foolish by being off with a bad back for the next few weeks.

How important is bed rest in the acute attack?

Very important, and as soon as possible. If your attack occurs at work, you may be in the kind of job where you can't just get up and leave. But as soon as it's practical, get home and get off your feet, to stop gravity from pressing down onto those sore joints or discs, because that pressure can trigger muscle spasms. Stay put, even for a few days, until the acute phase has subsided.

Any advice about the best way to lie in bed?

As I have said, there is no one best way. Adopt whatever position feels most comfortable. If the pain has been bad on forward bending, try lying on your stomach, as a temporary measure. If your back pain originates from a disc, even ten or fifteen minutes of lying on your stomach and arching your back slightly can make all the difference in getting rid of that spasm.

When your back pain originates in the spinal facet joints and arching backward increases your discomfort and pain, you should obviously get yourself into a position where you are hunched forward, to take the stress off those sore joints. Curl up in the fetal position with a pillow between your knees. Most people prefer a fat pillow, but try several to find the size you like best. Or lie on your back or your side and use the pelvic tilt, gently thrusting your hips forward to reduce the arch in your back. Whatever position you use, the important thing is to stay in bed and get up as little as possible.

What do you do next?

I try to relieve the pain through the use of a counter-irritant. Ice seems to work better for me at the moment, but heat and cold are both counter-irritants, and so they're both capable of reducing the pain. You should discover for yourself which one works best for you. Sometimes even alternating an ice pack and a hot-water bottle can be effective.

What about a hot bath, then, or a cold shower?

A cold shower would certainly take your mind off your back pain, but too much concentrated cold can actually increase the muscle spasm and increase your problem. I suggest you try a hot shower instead. Standing in the shower with one foot up on a ledge or low stool may be just the thing to relax your back. The sitting posture in a bathtub may put too much strain on your spine and offset the benefit of the heat. Also, a lot of people with bad backs find that getting in and out of a bathtub is so uncomfortable that the benefits aren't worth the effort.

People who have access to more modern conveniences will find that a whirlpool bath or a hot-tub can provide all the benefits of a hot bath without requiring you to curl up in a way that might put a needless load on your discs. Being able to stretch out in a hot-tub or lie with your back to the jet in a whirlpool is certainly excellent emergency treatment, if you have one of those facilities at hand.

Whatever form of bathing you choose, remember that you aren't your normal self, and if possible you should have someone there to help you in and out of the shower or tub, to avoid an accident.

Are there other effective counter-irritants besides heat and cold?

Yes. Liniment often provides relief, although you should recognize that neither the liniment nor the heat it produces actually reaches the muscle. By causing a burning sensation on the skin, liniment helps block the pain signals from deeper inside the body.

What other remedies are worth trying?

Gentle stretching often helps. The order of action is: rest your back, ice it (or heat it), and then stretch it. By stretching I mean just moving your back gently, in the directions that are comfortable. If bending in one direction causes pain, don't bend that way; try the other direction. If both directions hurt, wait a few hours before trying again.

You may actually produce comfort with gentle, repetitive movement in the direction that causes pain. In other words, start off by doing the things that are least painful. Then when you've recovered some mobility, cautiously try doing the things that hurt. For example, if forward bending hurts, gently bend forward to the point of discomfort and then stop. Then repeat that movement several times. If the movement is making the pain worse, don't persist. But if it isn't any worse, or if you begin to notice some slight improvement, keep it up. Spend a few minutes gently – and I emphasize gently – repeating the movement. Rest for a while, then try it again later on. Do this perhaps eight or ten times a day for a few days.

What about medication?

Having done all the right things during the first stage of your attack – and those are by far the most important counter-measures you can take – you may gain additional benefit from a relaxant or an anti-inflammatory drug. If your doctor is already familiar with your back problem, you can probably arrange by telephone to have one of these medications prescribed for you on an emergency basis. But be aware that they don't always work. There's just no guarantee. I find there is about a fifty-fifty chance of relief, whether you are taking anti-inflammatories or muscle relaxants. And, by the way, the drugs aren't just *back* muscle relaxants – they relax your whole body. I usually refer to them as "people relaxants."

What about pain killers?

Pain killers may help you get over the worst of it, although they can be surprisingly ineffective with acute back pain. Remember, they do nothing to alter the actual mechanism of the spasm. They simply dull your perception of pain. That effect may be welcome, but it might be unwise for you to take a strong medication in some circumstances. It could present a risk, for instance, if you took something at work and then tried to drive home. In that situation, you're better off just toughing things out until you're safely through the door.

What about a good belt of brandy – or whatever?

Alcohol can be helpful, if you're normally a moderate drinker. I'd hate to think that anyone would use a pain attack as an excuse to go home and get drunk. But a couple of drinks, in a controlled situation, and combined with bed rest, may help to relieve the tension and the anxiety that go along with the spasm.

Is it a matter of choosing between alcohol and medication? Or is it okay to take both?

It's usually a good idea to make it one or the other and not mix the two. On their own, anti-inflammatories and alcohol are both inclined to upset your stomach. So a dose of each could cause stomach problems you don't need, especially when you're already in pain. If you're taking strong pain relievers or relaxants, they'll cloud your thinking and make you drowsy, and alcohol will only accentuate that effect. That's not necessarily a bad thing, if it helps you sleep. But I am always concerned about the risk of becoming dependent on alcohol or any other addictive substance.

How long does an acute attack usually last?

Most attacks originating in the facet joints will be gone within a few days – two weeks at the most. The pain may be replaced by a dull ache or discomfort that may last for several weeks, but the acute episode is usually gone within a matter of days.

Do some attacks last longer?

Yes. If you have an attack of pain from a bulging disc, it will probably last four or five weeks. And it's a different kind of attack. Not everyone responds in exactly the same way, of course, but generally speaking disc pain tends to come on more slowly than facet pain. Often patients with disc problems will tell me, "I did something to my back in the morning, and by that night it was much worse. By the next day I couldn't move."

What's the shortest period I can hope for?

Just minutes to hours. If you act quickly and manage to beat it, you could be out of the acute attack before the day is through. At best you will have truly minimized it. It is well worth developing the skills to get around those painful episodes and continue to function normally.

But remember what I said earlier: *without exception, every single acute episode will end.* Furthermore, the original source of trouble will resolve. With time, the body repairs worn joints and bulging discs, and only the muscle pain remains to be treated.

I've heard of backache sufferers who got relief by having chiropractors manipulate their spines. Is that worth trying?

By all means, as long as your problem has been accurately diagnosed and you know that your low-back pain is originating in a facet joint or a disc. In that case, manipulation is safe and may provide relief from acute muscle spasm. But if your problem is caused by direct nerve pressure, manipulation can actually make matters worse.

What are the chances that nerve pressure is the source of my pain?

Irritation and pain caused by something pressing directly on the nerve occur in only about 10 percent of all cases of common backache. That statistic alone means low-back manipulation is usually safe. And when properly employed, the treatment should bring prompt relief. Manipulation is not one of those routines where you have to feel worse before you feel better.

Would you recommend seeing a chiropractor?

I don't object to your going to a chiropractor for treatment of an attack of back pain, as long as your condition is properly defined before any manipulation is attempted.

Do I need a doctor to diagnose my problem? Can't a chiropractor do that?

He will certainly try. Some chiropractors are good diagnosticians; many others are not. I'd want to feel confident that my chiropractor could detect nerve pressure and, if he found it, would not attempt manipulation. If you're not that confident about a chiropractor's diagnostic abilities, I'd suggest you get a second opinion before proceeding. I am not opposed to chiropractic treatment, but I do have certain reservations, which I will discuss later.

Is a chiropractor the only one who can provide relief by manipulation?

No. In my own practice I usually refer patients to trained physical therapists (or, as we say in Canada, physiotherapists), who are well qualified to perform manipulation. A massage therapist can also provide temporary relief by relaxing the muscle spasm, to get you through that crucial first stage.

What is the attack like if the pain is caused by direct nerve irritation?

There may be a sudden onset of pain, and typically it will be felt more in the leg than in the back. The leg pain may last for a considerable length of time and even be associated with weakness in certain groups of muscles.

If the pain runs into my leg, does that mean I must have a pinched nerve?

No, I didn't say that. All types of back pain can radiate into the leg, and most do. But you can use this test: say to yourself, "I am allowed to complain of only one pain. Which one will it be – the pain in my leg or the pain in my back?" If you choose the leg, there is a good chance that the pain is caused by nerve irritation. If you choose your back or your buttocks, you're probably in the

90 percent group – the people who have either facet or disc pain. You could try one other test to determine the cause of the pain in your leg. Pain in the toes is generally associated with direct nerve pressure. But be careful: we're talking here only about *leg pain* – not the numbness or tingling feelings that so often accompany an attack.

When you describe a disc pain attack as lasting for weeks, are you saying the person will be completely immobilized that whole time?

No. What it means is that after you've come to terms with the initial episode, you will have to rely heavily for some time on all the skills I hope you have learned, or will learn from this book, for dealing with your back. And, depending on the particular situation, I might recommend using a brace.

But aren't you on record somewhere as saying braces aren't a good idea?

Not exactly. I've always maintained that a brace is no substitute for muscle control and exercise. But in the short term, right after an acute attack, a brace may be the only thing that will get you up and around.

And once you are mobile, you should use all those tricks we've talked about here and in Chapter 1. Move slowly with care and grace. Don't make any sudden movements. Use the right seating. Make use of a foot-rest, and so on.

Is this one of those situations where the person's attitude is also important?

Definitely. Fear is your worst enemy. If you're constantly afraid of having another attack, or if you're worried that the present attack will never end, you're bound to be tense. And that tension, of course, will perpetuate the very spasm that is causing the pain. Once you know how to cope with an attack, and once you realize it will subside, you have no reason to be afraid, and you stand a far better chance of recovering quickly.

That sounds very positive – as long as the person has begun a proper program of back care. But what about people who haven't started?

Well, if you've just had an acute attack of pain, this is not the time to begin a long-range program of back care, including daily exercises. But perhaps the attack will serve as your motivation to get started as soon as you're back to normal. That's the best preventive medicine there is for bad backs.

Will regular exercise actually guarantee that you'll never have another attack?

There are no guarantees. Even the best automobile drivers have accidents. But certainly with the right exercise program you will substantially increase the odds in your favor.

3. WHY BACKS GET SORE

When I first wrote about the common causes of backache, I focused on the three principal sources of the pain: a worn facet joint, a bulging disc, and a pinched nerve. Recently, increasing numbers of back patients have been asking about a "new" condition called spinal stenosis, as though it were something doctors had just discovered.

In fact, the importance of an abnormally narrow spinal canal as a cause of pain has been recognized, at least by back specialists, for a generation or more. Its relationship to bulging discs was described in 1953 by Schlesinger and Taveras. In 1954 a Dutch surgeon named Verbiest made the significant observation that structural narrowing of the spinal canal alone could produce nerve-root compression.

In *The Back Doctor*, first published in 1980, I chose not to discuss spinal stenosis as an independent entity but to consider it merely a variation of the pinched nerve syndrome, which indeed it is. Since then, however, advancing medical knowledge and public concern have combined to convince me that spinal stenosis warrants separate classification, partly because of its distinctive characteristics and partly because the very act of singling it out in this way should help to make it more widely understood.

As a result, readers familiar with the contents of *The Back Doctor* may be especially interested to discover that, in this chapter, as I review and elaborate on the conditions responsible for common back pain, I refer not just to the three basic causes described in my first book, but to four. I hope that people who are anxious to know more about spinal stenosis will find their questions answered clearly and completely.

———————

What, exactly, causes a person's back to ache?

There are dozens of possible causes, but let's begin by talking about the causes of almost 90 percent of all cases of common backache, which is the affliction most people will want to know about. The basic problem can be summed up in three simple words: wear and tear, and age.

Wear and tear occurs in various forms over the years, often through nothing more than ordinary everyday activity. It affects the two principal parts of your spine: the little drum-shaped bones called vertebrae and the small, oval pads that separate and cushion them, called discs. Because of the way your spine is constructed, the vertebrae and discs in the lower part of your back carry the heaviest loads and are consequently subjected to the most wear and tear.

Each drum-shaped vertebra has a tunnel along its posterior edge and three wing-like parts protruding outward around that tunnel. A vertebra also has four specialized projections – two pointing upward and two downward – capped with cartilage: a smooth, slippery substance that allows easy movement. Each pair of upward projections interlocks with the pair of downward projections on the adjacent vertebra, forming two knuckle-sized joints called spinal facet joints, or simply facets. These joints are able to bear some of your body's weight, but their main function is to control movement, so that you won't bend or twist your back further than it should go.

Sometimes, as a person ages, a disc will dry out and flatten so much that the two joint surfaces above it will bear down and jam against the two joint surfaces below. That extra pressure within the two facet joints begins to wear away the cartilage covering the bones. This action roughens the surfaces and leads to pain in the joints, a very common cause of backache I call Type One back pain.

Type Two originates in the discs, which normally contain a jelly that helps them serve as cushions, not merely "spacers" between vertebrae. A healthy disc is an excellent hydraulic shock-absorber, although it does not contain any free liquid but rather a fluid-retaining gel. You couldn't puncture a disc with a needle and expect it to leak.

In a young disc, that soft nucleus functions to protect the spine. As a person reaches the mid-teens, the nucleus starts to slowly dry out. Through the years, the disc, losing some of its "cushiony" quality, flattens down in the center and bulges out around the edges. Imagine a round air-cushion half full of air. If you placed it on the floor and stepped on the center of it, the edges of the cushion would bulge out and might even pop open. That's about what happens with a bulging disc. As the shell of the disc spreads beyond its normal diameter, it stretches and frays. The central jelly, now rather hard and lumpy, may be pushed out through a split in the shell.

The outer portion of the disc is pain-sensitive, and if part of it bulges too far out of shape or tears, you will feel Type Two pain.

I think many people believe almost all backache comes from a pinched nerve.

Many people do believe that, while, in fact, Types One and Two are far more common. The pinched nerve is the cause of backache in only one out of every ten patients I see.

Many people also believe that backache caused by a pinched nerve is inevitably more severe than backache from the other two common causes. But that's not necessarily true either. The intensity of pain depends on the severity of local muscle spasm, a feature common to all three types; the amount of inflammation present; the degree of wear in the facet or disc; and the patient's individual response to pain. That last factor is something I will talk more about later.

In Type Three pain, a nerve is being pressed or irritated by a bulging disc, or, when the disc ruptures, by some of the nucleus that has squeezed out through a tear in the shell. This pinching generally occurs at a point where the nerve passes over the back corner of the disc on its way out of the spinal canal. If the disc ruptures, there are only two likely causes of nerve pain: the direct pressure I just mentioned, and an inflammatory reaction in the nerve caused by the jelly from inside the disc – one of nature's unwanted chemical spills.

Discs, however, are not the only source of pressure on the nerves. Nerve irritation is also a part of Type Four back pain, spinal stenosis.

As I mentioned, your spine has a passage called the spinal canal, which runs down through the back of each vertebra. It contains an elaborate system of nerve tissue known as the spinal cord, which is actually an extension of your brain. The spinal cord ends just below the level of your twelfth rib, and the spinal canal in the low back contains nothing but the nerves that run on down to the legs. This complex tangle has the name *cauda equina* or "horse's tail." A pair of nerves from the cord or from the *cauda equina* leaves the canal at every level through small openings on either side of the spine between adjacent vertebrae.

In some people's spines one or more of those openings or part of the lower canal itself is abnormally narrow – too narrow for the *cauda equina* or the roots to pass through comfortably. Like a shoe that's too tight for your foot, the narrow passage exerts pressure on the nerves. That condition is what we call spinal stenosis.

Is there some way for me to determine on my own whether my problem is common backache?

Yes, you can assess your own symptoms and conduct certain tests, which I'll describe in a moment. But first, it's important to make sure your pain is originating in your back. Pain along the spine doesn't always come from the back. Kidney pain, for example, is usually felt in the low back and in one flank and can be extremely severe. Another frequent source of confusion is pain in the hip, so you may want to try this little test:

Lie on your back and draw one knee up to your chest. Does that cause pain in your groin? If so, you may have hip trouble.

Now keep your knee bent and gently turn your lower leg outward. If that also causes pain in your groin and perhaps down the front of your thigh to your knee, the cause, again, may be in your hip. If neither movement causes pain, your hip is probably not to blame.

Is there a test to rule out injury to the back?

You don't need a test for that. If your back has been injured severely enough to cause serious structural damage, you will remember the incident: an airplane crash, a fall off a building, a major sports accident, that kind of thing. A healthy back is too rugged to be injured by minor bumping or an injudicious bit of bending or stretching.

Then what about disease as a cause of my back pain?

First, most diseases causing back pain also produce symptoms in so many parts of your body that you wouldn't consider yourself a backache victim, and you wouldn't be looking for answers in a book about backs.

Second, you can be fairly certain that your problem is not caused by a disease of the spine if you can answer "yes" to four questions:

1. Does your back feel better after a good rest?
2. Even if you have recurring attacks in rapid succession, do you usually recover from each acute episode within a few weeks?
3. When your back is bothering you, are you free of other symptoms: weight loss, skin rashes, fever, joint pain in your fingers, toes, hips, or knees?
4. Considering your age and physical condition, once the pain has subsided, does the movement in your back return to normal? Remember to take into account the fact that after a few weeks of rest and inactivity, most backs will stiffen up. You may require a little time and effort to regain your normal flexibility.

"Yes" answers to all four questions virtually ensure that your back pain is not caused by any disease. Even one or two "no" answers are not definite indication of a specific illness. Statistically, it is still far more likely that your problem is common backache – that is, Type One, Two, Three, or Four.

What are the symptoms of Type One and Type Two back pain?

If you have typical Type One pain, your description might go like this [with variations described in square brackets]:

Each attack begins with a minor incident or nothing at all. In my last incident, I simply bent over to pick up the lawn rake [golf ball, small grandchild]. Instantly, I had a flash of sharp pain in my back, which almost took my breath away. I couldn't move. The pain was worse when I tried to stand up straight, and it eased off a little when I bent forward.

My pain was mainly in my low back, although there was [sometimes but not necessarily] pain in my buttocks and down the back of my leg[s] as far as the knee[s]. I had no pain in my lower legs or feet. If you asked me to pinpoint my problem, I would say the most painful area was the top of my buttocks. I've had other attacks where the pain wasn't so severe but it always starts suddenly and stops me from going on with what I am doing. I know that if I try to arch my back the pain will get worse.

I get the same problem about two or three times a year. If I rest for a few days and don't aggravate the pain, it goes away completely within two weeks [as soon as four or five days]. Usually I can do anything I want between attacks and feel no pain [but I'm always aware of some discomfort that makes me a little nervous].

If you have typical Type Two pain, you might describe your problem this way:

My first attack began when I slipped on a patch of ice, twisted my back but didn't fall [when I found myself holding the whole 200-pound box after my partner suddenly let go].

Like the Type One patient, I've had other attacks following some minor lifting [sudden twists, hockey game, golf swing] but my symptoms are not quite the same. I feel something go [give, pull] in my back. I wouldn't describe it as pain but I know I've done something. At first it's just discomfort. The pain builds up over several hours [a day or two] until it is really severe. It recedes within a few weeks after that, but it doesn't disappear. Instead, it lingers on. One time it was just a nagging backache [another time it was really intense].

TYPE ONE (FACET JOINT PAIN)

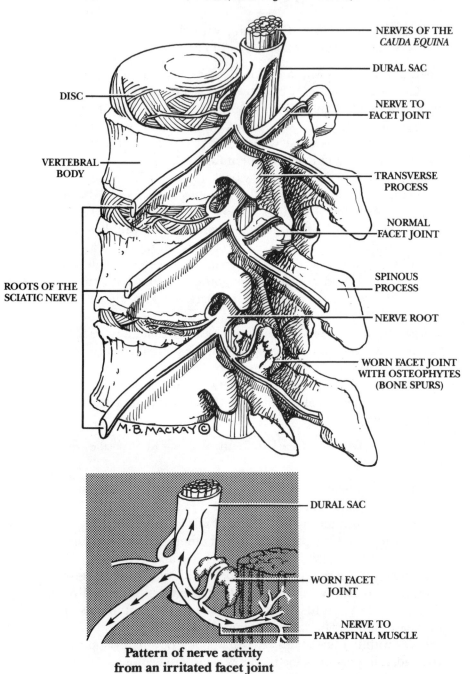

Pattern of nerve activity
from an irritated facet joint

The Type One patient said it hurt to bend backward and felt good to bend forward. I have exactly the opposite problem, and so when I'm active again after an attack, I stand up as straight as I can, and I avoid bending forward or lifting anything.

My pain is mainly in my low back, but I can feel it as well in my buttocks and upper legs — pretty much, I gather, the same as the Type One pain.

The worst part of my problem is that, although an acute attack will be gone in four or five weeks [two or three weeks], it can take me as long as three months [six months] to recover completely.

If you are one of the unfortunates who have a combination of Type One *and* Type Two, you might add this comment:

I have kept a record of my attacks and their duration, and I find that not all my attacks begin the same way or last the same amount of time. I have had acute, short-term attacks interspersed with longer-lasting ones.

Is the problem more serious if it combines Type One with Type Two?

No. But, compared to either type alone, the source of the pain is harder to locate. It's important to note that the wear of normal aging takes place in joints and discs alike, so both areas are usually affected even though only one may cause trouble.

If these descriptions have left you uncertain whether you have Type One or Type Two pain, you might like to perform a few simple tests, which will do you no harm, although they may cause momentary discomfort. Of course I don't recommend that you undertake any testing of this kind while you are still in acute pain. Wait until the attack begins to subside and you feel confident about making unfamiliar movements.

Type One pain increases when you arch backwards to look up. The pain is felt mainly in the back and it radiates downward no further than the knees.

Type Two pain is worse when you bend forward and, again, it is back not leg pain that discourages further movement.

These are positive tests. When one of them produces typical

TYPE TWO (DISC PAIN)

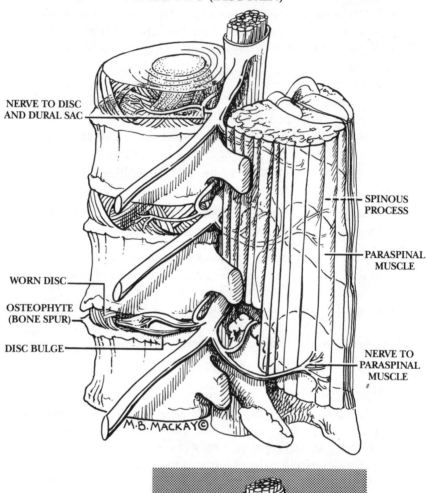

NERVE TO DISC
AND DURAL SAC

SPINOUS
PROCESS

PARASPINAL
MUSCLE

WORN DISC

OSTEOPHYTE
(BONE SPUR)

DISC BULGE

NERVE TO
PARASPINAL
MUSCLE

M.B.MACKAY©

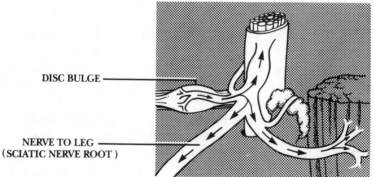

DISC BULGE

NERVE TO LEG
(SCIATIC NERVE ROOT)

**Pattern of nerve activity
from a bulging disc**

pain, we know immediately where the problem lies. A negative test helps confirm that a certain condition does *not* exist. This next test is designed to help you rule out the possibility that your problem is Type Three, a pinched nerve.

As you lie on your back, try to lift one leg with the knee straight. If you can't lift your leg alone, have someone help, gently. Lifting your leg may increase your back pain, but this is not significant, since this movement can aggravate either Type One or Type Two discomfort. The pain to check for is pain radiating down the leg, particularly below the knee and into the foot and toes. If it's Type Three, the pain should occur before the leg is lifted two-thirds of the way to the vertical. Pain occurring after the leg is lifted above that height is generally the result of tight muscles and poor flexibility.

If this test is negative – that is, if you can accomplish the two-thirds lift without pain radiating into your leg – you can conclude with fair certainty that you do not have Type Three pain, and that, as a victim of common backache, your problem must be Type One, Type Two, or a combination of both.

The back pain in Type Four trouble is either from the joints (Type One) or from the discs (Type Two). Although the spinal stenosis may produce pressure on a nerve, the pattern of leg pain differs considerably from Type Three.

What are the symptoms if my problem is Type Three, that is a nerve pinched by a bulging disc?

For a quick grasp of Type Three symptoms, refer back to the description of Type Two. All the symptoms you see there apply to Type Three; but there is one substantial difference. A typical Type Three patient might describe it this way:

My problem is not really my back but my leg. My leg pain is far worse than my back pain, and it doesn't stop at my knees; it radiates into my lower legs [and in some cases, into my feet and toes].

TYPE THREE (PINCHED NERVE)

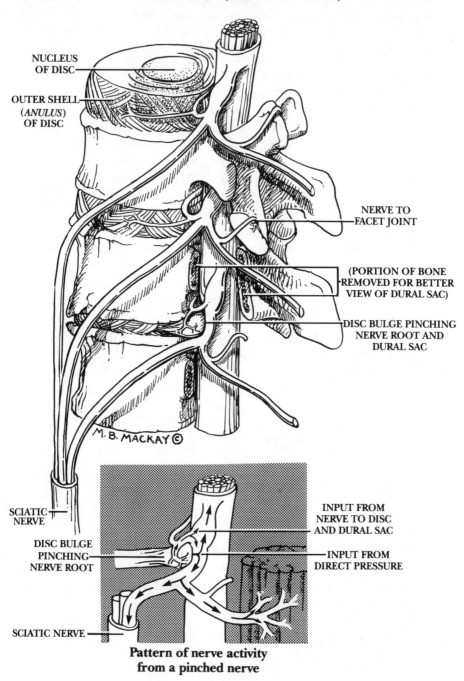

NUCLEUS OF DISC

OUTER SHELL (*ANULUS*) OF DISC

NERVE TO FACET JOINT

(PORTION OF BONE REMOVED FOR BETTER VIEW OF DURAL SAC)

DISC BULGE PINCHING NERVE ROOT AND DURAL SAC

M. B. MACKAY ©

SCIATIC NERVE

DISC BULGE PINCHING NERVE ROOT

SCIATIC NERVE

INPUT FROM NERVE TO DISC AND DURAL SAC

INPUT FROM DIRECT PRESSURE

Pattern of nerve activity from a pinched nerve

Besides straight-leg raising, what other tests can I do to check for Type Three trouble?

Pressure on a nerve usually causes irritation but no loss of normal function. In rare instances when the nerve does lose its ability to conduct messages in an orderly fashion, there are three groups of tests we conduct: for muscle power, reflexes, and sensory ability. The examinations, in order of their reliability and significance, are:

A two-part test for muscle power.
Part 1: Stand erect and try to raise yourself into a tip-toe position, that is by raising your heels so you're standing on the balls of your feet. Raise and lower yourself ten times this way, on both feet at once and then on each foot separately. The pain may restrict your movement, but if your muscle power is normal you should nevertheless be able to perform this action.
Part 2: Stand with your feet comfortably apart. Now raise your toes and arches as high off the floor as you can and see whether you can walk that way, with your weight entirely on your heels. It's not a comfortable position at the best of times, but, disregarding the way it may aggravate your back pain, you should able to walk as well this way now as you ever could.

If you passed both parts of the test, your nerve activity to the muscles is probably normal.

A test of your knee and ankle reflexes. What you are trying to find out here is not whether your reflexes are strong or weak but whether they have been changed by your spinal problem. It's significant, for instance, if you find that your once-strong reflexes are now noticeably weaker, or if they have become weaker in one leg than in the other. If your reflexes are normal, your back condition has not affected the function in the nerves that supply the reflex action.
Knee reflex test: Sit in a chair of normal height and dangle one knee over the other. With a heavy object (such as a moderately thick book), tap the exposed knee sharply but not too severely in the soft area below the kneecap. (Or have someone do the tapping for you.) If the tapping is done properly and your reflex is normal, your leg will kick upward in a sudden,

involuntary motion. If you do not get that reaction the first time, try several taps before drawing any conclusions. Now switch to repeat the test on the other knee. If both legs react with the same involuntary kick, the nerve that supplies that reflex is probably normal.

Ankle reflex test: Sit down in an ordinary chair, remove your shoes, and lay the side of one calf over the other knee so that the ankle and foot project out to one side. Now, in the same sort of action you used on your knee, rap your Achilles' tendon – that thick tendon at the back of your ankle, right above the heel. If you conduct the test correctly, your foot should jerk downwards. Since this is a harder test to conduct on yourself than the knee reflex test, you may prefer to have someone test your ankle reflexes for you. In that case, you can adopt a different position: kneel on the chair with your ankles hanging free and have the other person tap gently on one tendon and then the other. Once several reactions have occurred, consider whether they are more or less the same for both ankles. If so, it is unlikely your nerve function in that area is impaired.

A test of your legs' sensory ability: The objective here is to determine whether certain parts of your legs or feet have lost sensation. You are trying to discover whether you still have the ability to feel the brief flash of pain you normally get from a pinprick in the skin. Note that this test ranks third in order of significance and reliability. That's because the area of skin served by a single nerve is quite variable and because only you can report on the finding. Your muscular performance and your reflexes could be observed by others as well as yourself, but no companion or doctor – even someone who conducts the test for you – can record the extent of the pain you feel (or don't feel).

For this test, bare your feet and lower legs, equip yourself with a safety pin, and sit down. Now reach down and use the open safety pin in a short, jabbing motion to test three areas on your feet and legs. First, prick the top of the big toe and along the inner side of the foot. Now prick the opposite side of the same foot, from the little toe down the outside edge. Third, prick a spot anywhere on the calf along the inside of the leg.

Now repeat this procedure on the other foot and leg. If every one of these pinpricks produces typical pain, there's nothing wrong with the nerves' ability to conduct normal impulses from the skin.

If the results of these three groups of tests have all been negative, you have ruled out nerve damage caused by Type Three or Type Four back trouble. Your problem, in all likelihood, is Type One or Type Two pain or, at the very most, Type Three pain with only nerve-root irritation.

I guess that brings us back to Type Four pain – spinal stenosis. How does it develop?

As I said earlier, spinal stenosis is a condition in which the passage containing the large collection of nerves at the bottom of the spine, the *cauda equina*, is abnormally narrow. "Stenosis" just means "narrowing." It's a condition that can be either congenital or acquired.

In a congenital case, the person is born with a small spinal canal that is triangular in cross section instead of the normal five-sided shape. This abnormal size and shape may exist in just a short segment or it may extend throughout the whole lumbar canal. The condition will remain undetected unless the amount of narrowing is enough for the nerves to start feeling the squeeze.

Acquired spinal stenosis will develop when the volume of the spinal canal is reduced by a chronically bulging disc or the normal extra growth of bone that occurs in the spine with age. Of course, stenosis may occur through a combination of congenital and acquired causes – a narrow canal made even narrower by a bulging disc or new bone.

Spinal stenosis sounds like a very serious problem.

Actually the stenosis, in itself, is not the problem. Having a narrow spinal canal is no more painful than, say, having narrow feet. The problem arises when the lack of space interferes with the normal functioning of a nerve. Every symptomatic case of spinal stenosis involves pressure on a nerve, and so in a broad sense, it's like Type Three back pain. But the nature of that pressure is different, and so are the symptoms.

TYPE FOUR (SPINAL STENOSIS)

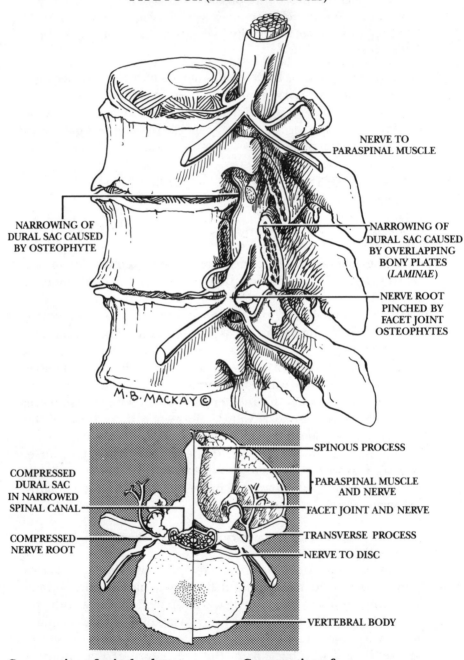

NERVE TO
PARASPINAL MUSCLE

NARROWING OF
DURAL SAC CAUSED
BY OSTEOPHYTE

NARROWING OF
DURAL SAC CAUSED
BY OVERLAPPING
BONY PLATES
(*LAMINAE*)

NERVE ROOT
PINCHED BY
FACET JOINT
OSTEOPHYTES

M.B. MACKAY©

COMPRESSED
DURAL SAC
IN NARROWED
SPINAL CANAL

COMPRESSED
NERVE ROOT

SPINOUS PROCESS

PARASPINAL MUSCLE
AND NERVE

FACET JOINT AND NERVE

TRANSVERSE PROCESS

NERVE TO DISC

VERTEBRAL BODY

Cross section of spinal column
with stenosis

Cross section of
normal spinal column

In what way are stenosis symptoms different?

Without enough room in the spinal canal, the nerves of the *cauda equina* can't get the extra nourishment they need to supply active muscles. This additional energy normally comes from an increase in the blood supply to the nerves, and a tight fit prevents the blood vessels from expanding to carry the load. At rest, the system manages to keep up with the demand, but as soon as the leg muscles start to work, the nerves are in trouble. In what I call the language of Doctor, this condition is known as *cauda equina* claudication. It occurs only when the narrowing or stenosis is sufficient to interfere with the blood supply to the "horse's tail" or to exiting nerve roots.

If you have typical Type Four pain you might describe your problem this way:

> My back isn't really my problem, it's my legs. And they only cause trouble when I walk. After about ten minutes [a quarter mile, two blocks, a walk down the mall] they get all rubbery [dead, heavy, cold, numb] and I have to stop. If I can sit down for a few [ten to twenty] minutes, my legs feel better, and I can start walking again.
>
> I've noticed I can get relief faster if I sit with one leg drawn up [body bent forward, leaning to one side].
>
> I've tried the Type One, Two, and Three tests. My back hurts more if I bend backward [forward, or doesn't hurt at all]. The rest of the tests indicated no problems.

If the pain is caused by stenosis, does it ever come on as a sudden attack?

No. In cases where the disc is the culprit, the stenosis develops gradually as the disc bulges and begins taking up space in the nerve canal. Unlike the fairly sudden, acute bulging-disc conditions I call Type Two and Type Three pain, this is a slow and subtle impingement on the nerve. Consequently, the person doesn't experience the acute onset of pain that comes with a ruptured disc or the chemical reaction that occurs when the jelly escapes. Instead, the pain develops gradually over time.

In the other form of acquired stenosis, where bony growth is to blame, the narrowing often develops from nature's attempt to overcome facet, or Type One, pain. As you'll remember, I described how the flattening of a disc forces the pair of facet joints to come under increasing pressure. At first, the slippery cartilage surfaces are worn away, producing facet pain. Eventually they become jammed so tightly together that the rubbing stops. And now that the joint is stiff, there is less pain because there's less movement. At that stage, the body begins reshaping the bones of the spine to suit the new conditions.

The body reshapes the spine? How?

Two ways. First, by forming little bony projections or spurs called osteophytes, which help stabilize the joints and disc spaces; osteophytes can do this by growing out from adjacent vertebrae and forming a bridge of bone, which fuses the joint or encloses the disc. And second, the body reshapes the spine by removing other parts of the bone to leave ample room for the exiting nerve roots. When this process is complete, the affected segment of the spine is fused just as securely as it would be if the fusion had been performed by the finest surgeon in the world. The joint is now truly pain-free – but it has also ceased being a joint.

Does this stiffening of the joints and discs immobilize the spine?

No. The amount of stiffness that occurs with fusing one or two levels of the spine is not as serious as you might imagine, and there are certainly many people with stiff backs who can move well enough to participate in a number of sports. You won't be as flexible at sixty as you were at sixteen, but that needn't stop you from leading an active life.

What do osteophytes look like?

Osteophytes have many shapes. Some are just bony lumps that tend to form around worn joints. You can see them often in old people's fingers, in the joints nearest the fingertips. Those cartoons of witches with knobby fingers are exaggerations of a real condition that affects older people as osteophytes form around various joints of their bodies.

Then having those little spurs – osteophytes – in your spine is normal for most people?

Yes. Their growth is normal, part of aging, and the body's regular process of repairing itself.

Do osteophytes ever hurt?

Not usually. People often get upset when their doctors point out this condition on their X-rays. They assume that these bone spurs (which are sometimes described incorrectly as calcium deposits) are a cause of pain – but this is not so. In the early stages when there are periods of rapid growth, osteophytes can be tender, but they don't cause pain.

Then osteophytes don't have to be removed?

Not unless they are causing trouble. More often, they're serving a good purpose. By enlarging the surfaces of the joint, the bone spurs reduce the load on any single point and help to decrease Type One pain.

Spurs also form around the edges of dried-out discs, protecting them from being squashed further. They poke out from the sides of the vertebral bodies like little fingers. In some cases they extend up or down, partly enclosing the disc space and bringing one vertebra into contact with its neighbor, creating a certain amount of stability.

But osteophytes in the spine do cause trouble sometimes?

Yes – they sometimes bring on Type Four back pain. Once in a while a spur that has developed to protect a joint from increased pressure will perform a disservice instead by growing into the spinal canal and squeezing against the nerve root that exits just beside the joint. Doctors refer to this condition as bony entrapment.

Is there any way I can test myself for Type Four pain?

As we've seen, Type Four pain is due to nerve compression similar to Type Three but without the acute onset and chemical reaction. For this reason the tests for muscle power, reflexes, and sensation are usually normal in Type Four trouble *except* when the nerves are working hard and running short of blood. If you suspect you have this type of back problem, go for a walk or do whatever you normally do to bring on the pain. Then, as the attack subsides, perform all the Type Three test maneuvers. This is called a provocative test. If there is any loss of normal nerve conduction – and usually there is *not* – it will be brought out under stress.

Pain may be produced on backward bending (indicating Type One backache) or on forward bending (indicating Type Two). Both types are possible, but pain on arching backward is more common for people suffering with spinal stenosis.

Can spinal stenosis be cured by surgery?

Often it can, in an operation that removes the protruding bone or chronically bulging disc and relieves pressure on the nerve. The operation is called a spinal decompression. As you might suppose, surgery is likely to produce the best results when the narrowing is limited to one or two levels. The more levels involved, the more difficult the surgery and the less likely we are to have a good long-term result.

It's important for patients to understand that we operate because there is nerve-root compression, not simply because we detect a narrow passage.

What if surgery isn't feasible for a person with spinal stenosis – I mean, with nerve-root compression? Are there other kinds of treatment?

Certainly. The right exercises can help a lot. So can better postural habits. But even if surgery is recommended, a person with spinal stenosis should first get started on an exercise program. In most cases patients need flexion (that is, forward bending) exercises; although extension (backward bending) exercises sometimes help. Proper posture is important because it helps keep the spinal canal in the best possible alignment to offer the nerves all the room available.

At the time spinal stenosis is diagnosed as the cause of pressure on the *cauda equina,* or on individual nerve roots, the doctor has no way of assessing the possible benefit to be gained from exercise. Exercise alone may be a sufficient remedy. On the other hand, the doctor and patient may find that in spite of their best efforts, the narrowing is so extreme that relief is possible only through a spinal decompression. Even so, the exercise can do no harm, and obviously it's advisable to try for the maximum benefit without surgery.

Is there a danger, though, of putting off the surgery until it's too late?

No. As long as your condition isn't noticeably getting worse, surgery can be done at any time. The doctor's classic line, "If only you'd come to see me sooner I could have helped you," doesn't apply here. Obviously, if you're having severe pain you'll want to get rid of it as soon as you can. But if there's a good reason for delaying surgery, you can safely pick a time that suits you.

Recently I examined a man with severe spinal stenosis at two levels. In his case, surgery is definitely called for. But he's a busy man. He runs his own one-man company, supplying artificial flowers to florists. It's a seasonal business, and if he stops working during a peak period his company could go under.

The poor man can hardly get in and out of his truck, and so he is torn between the need to keep working and the need for surgery. His question is: "If I wait until next fall, will I have waited too long?"

Fortunately, I could tell him there is no harm in waiting. Since his condition shows no signs of growing worse, there is no reason why the operation can't be delayed for a few months. And in the interim he can try some exercises that might help reduce the pain.

Can surgery relieve Type Four pain even if the person is well on in years?

Oh, yes, it often can. One of my patients is a man in his mid-seventies whose stenosis was preventing him from pursuing his favorite pastime, square dancing. Whenever he danced he got pain in his legs and had to stop. I put him on a program of flexion exercises, and when I found that surgery was feasible I carried out a standard spinal decompression. Six months later he came back and told me with great satisfaction that he could now square dance two sets per evening. In his prime he would dance three sets, but now he was delighted to manage two. Whether stenosis patients have surgery or not, they must realize they are faced with an anatomical problem which may be improved upon but which in some cases cannot be fully corrected, and so they must settle for a few compromises.

Now that you have described the four types, have we covered all the sources of common backache?

No, but we have covered the primary causes. There are several important secondary factors, such as muscle spasm, segmental instability, torsion injury, and minor trauma. They are considered secondary not because they are less painful but because they usually arise from one of the primary causes.

How do muscle spasms fit into this pattern of common backache?

Spasms are very common but they are almost always caused by one of the four primary problems. When part of your spine is irritated or under tension, the muscles at the scene become alerted to the fact that a joint or a disc is in trouble and they tense up to protect the area while it is healing. Their reaction is often sudden and sharp, as it is, for instance, if you sprain a spinal joint. Unfortunately, those muscles may tense up so much that they become painful themselves. You recognize the reaction as a spasm or cramp, and it's the commonest way for muscles to become a source of back pain.

If a muscle is in spasm, it draws extra blood, thereby raising its own temperature. As we'll see later in our discussion of diagnostic tools, this extra heat can be readily detected by a technique called thermography.

When you speak of tension in this case, I presume you mean physical tension.

Not necessarily. Emotional tension can also cause muscle spasm. That's one reason why the psychological factor is often an important component of back pain. You may send one or several muscles into spasm either by tensing up *in fear* of physical back pain, or by tensing up *in response* to it. Either way, your emotions have triggered new or additional pain that otherwise would not have occurred. And as long as you keep reacting that way, you have a self-perpetuating problem.

Then how do you ever get over it?

The answer is easy to say and hard to do: relax. That's one reason why a short period of rest is so important early in an acute attack. But, however you treat it, sooner or later, the tension and pain will disappear as the underlying cause resolves and the muscle spasm relaxes.

What is segmental instability – and is it as frightening as it sounds?

It's hardly what you would call a desirable condition, but it isn't grounds for panic. A literal reading of the phrase tells you pretty much what's involved: a segment of the spine (and by that I mean the disc and facet joints that separate a pair of vertebrae) has a little too much play in it and is therefore unstable. It doesn't mean that your spine is about to collapse in a heap.

In practical terms, you may have trouble straightening up after bending forward. Instead of returning to an erect position in the normal way, you find yourself hitching to one side as you straighten up, as if you were coming up around an invisible post. When a normal spine straightens up, it unwinds from the bottom up in a precise sequence, so that the load – that is, the weight of your body – is transmitted in the most efficient way possible. When a segment of the spine is unstable, the system can't follow that sequence, and the load has to be handled in another, less efficient way.

What causes a segment to become unstable?

Usually it's just the wear and tear of aging in the low back. As a disc dries, squashes down, and bulges out, it loses its firm cushion effect and allows an abnormal degree of movement between the vertebrae above and below it. The facets must accept a greater amount of movement, and that strains the joint coverings. All this produces a little hitch as the spine attempts to move. Again, I stress that the abnormal movement is so slight that nothing will slip out of place, but it is enough to alter the way your spine behaves.

Is segmental instability painful?

Usually it is, and the pain may be different from simple facet or disc pain. Typically it takes the form of sudden sharp jabs, occurring when the person twists suddenly or straightens up from a forward-bent position. The pain is not necessarily felt at the site of the trouble. It often radiates into the top of the buttocks. The actual location of the problem can sometimes be determined by pressing sideways on the bony projections that you can feel along the spine under the surface of the skin. The area of instability may be tender, if not sore. Of course, local muscle spasm can give the same pattern of tenderness in the back, and for that reason the examination is of limited value.

Is there a satisfactory remedy for segmental instability?

Occasionally exercise to strengthen the muscles along the spine can give good relief. For greater degrees of instability the solution may be an operation in which the two adjacent vertebrae are fused together so that they function as a jointless unit. This operation has a high success ratio when the instability is found in only one segment. If several levels are unstable, surgery is more difficult and less likely to succeed.

A friend's young daughter went through a screening program at school and was found to have scoliosis. Naturally, her parents are quite upset.

The term scoliosis refers to an abnormal, side-to-side curve of the spine. Viewed from behind, the back should appear a straight line. The S-shaped curve of scoliosis can result from several conditions: abnormalities of spinal growth, certain neuro-muscular diseases, the extreme effects of wear and tear, and even, temporarily, the severe muscle spasm that can accompany Type Two or Type Three back pain. The term scoliosis, however, describes only the presence of the curve and says nothing about the cause.

I can understand how that girl's parents feel, but chances are they have nothing to worry about. Idiopathic scoliosis (the kind that results from abnormal growth in the spine) is found in about 5 percent of all children, and most cases are so mild that they require no medical attention whatever. Slight curves cause no complications or pain and are scarcely noticeable except to a physician or a nurse who is looking specifically for this condition. Parents are likely to notice only when they see their child wearing a bathing-suit or getting fitted in a clothing store.

Even most of the severe curves are no cause for alarm. They are usually painless, and they can be remedied in several ways if they are detected early. And, these days, most cases *are* detected early, either by family physicians or through scoliosis screening in our schools.

What causes idiopathic scoliosis?

The word "idiopathic," in Doctor, means "without cause." We know a lot about the condition but we don't know exactly why it happens. It is by far the commonest form of scoliosis – the type the public health people look for during the school screening programs. It develops around the age of puberty and is found more often in girls than in boys. For some unknown reason it almost always causes the upper spine to curve to the left. The curve is often associated with a rotation of the spine pushing the ribs backward on the right side of the chest and producing the typical hump. A child's susceptibility to the condition is related to hereditary factors, but researchers have yet to come up with ways of predicting or preventing it.

I've heard that scoliosis causes back pain. Isn't that true?

Surprisingly, idiopathic scoliosis doesn't usually cause pain. The incidence of common backache among people with scoliosis is about the same as for the population at large. And so when people with scoliosis come to me complaining of back pain, I explain that they have two problems: the back pain and the curvature, and each must be treated separately.

What's the treatment for scoliosis?

In most cases, none. Generally the curvature of the spine is so slight that people don't even know they have scoliosis unless it is detected by someone else. Those mild cases cause no difficulties of any kind – even in appearance.

A few youngsters have scoliosis that progresses rapidly during their teens, and they require treatment. Usually they wear braces during their growing years, to keep their spines in proper alignment, much the way you brace a plant to help it grow straight. If bracing is not sufficient, surgery may be required to straighten the back.

For the small percentage of patients who must undergo surgical correction, the process can be arduous. Occasionally, more than one operation is required, and the time in hospital can extend over many weeks. After surgery, the patient is usually required to wear a custom-fitted brace for several months until the fusion is complete. Although major surgery of this type is painful and the effect of repeated hospitalizations can disrupt a normal childhood, the end result with current operative techniques is generally excellent.

Does a scoliotic curve keep getting worse throughout a person's life?

Not very often. If the curve is slight or moderate, it stops progressing, even without medical intervention, once the person is fully grown. Sometimes a severe curve will continue to progress after maturity and require fusion; a brace is no use at that stage.

Some of the fear about scoliosis has arisen because of stories concerning the unusual extreme case that was neglected until it distorted the person's whole body. Or the fear may reflect someone's brief encounter with a child in the midst of a series of intimidating operations or suffering post-surgical complications. But thanks to our increased awareness and surgical skill, such cases are rare these days.

If idiopathic scoliosis is detected at an early stage, as happened with your friend's daughter, there is usually nothing to worry about. She probably won't need treatment of any kind. At most, she will need to have the curve corrected by bracing or, far less likely, by surgery. But one way or another, with modern management, she has little to fear from scoliosis.

You said earlier that some types of injuries are also considered secondary causes of backache. What types did you mean?

I make a distinction between two degrees of injury: on the one hand, a violent physical disruption of the spine – the kind of injury you might suffer in a high-speed automobile crash or by diving head first into a shallow swimming pool – and on the other hand, the degree of everyday strain that will bring on a pain attack because a facet joint or disc has already been made vulnerable through wear and tear. I consider this latter kind of injury to be a secondary factor because it arises out of one of those primary causes of common backache.

Although I keep pointing out that there's an important difference between "hurt," which suggests merely irritation resulting in temporary pain, and "harm," which indicates actual damage, sometimes it's hard for the back pain sufferer to tell them apart. If you walk barefoot on a beach and stub your toe on a rock, you may or may not consider it a serious injury. Even though it's terribly painful you know it's "just a stubbed toe" that will heal itself. Yet there may be an element of physical damage that can lead to annoying, long-term problems. The same principle applies when you sprain a facet joint.

But how would a sprain occur in a facet joint? People don't go around stubbing their spines.

You can wrench a spinal joint and cause an acute sprain by twisting your back violently or picking up a heavy load. The resulting Type One pain may come and go for months. Even though you have not damaged the joint, and it will eventually heal, it may cause you pain for so long that you come to believe the injury is permanent.

It's worth remembering that, compared to the joints in your

fingers or toes, a facet joint can withstand a considerable amount of punishment.

But with a spinal joint sprain, there is also a heavy emotional factor you don't usually find with, say, a sprained ankle. Because they don't understand much about their spines, many people are fearful of having anything happen "back there" and, often, they're terrified of permanent disability. Recognizing the emotional component, you can see how a relatively minor facet joint sprain can quickly become magnified into a major attack of back pain.

If the strain is severe enough, however, the joint may never recover fully from the damage and may remain slightly more susceptible to a new strain or injury, just as you might live out your life with a "trick knee" or weak ankle that was injured years before.

Does that mean that an old injury you've all but forgotten can remain dormant for years and then suddenly flare up in an attack of back pain?

No – that simply doesn't happen. If you're one of those people who have an old problem that flares up every so often, you'll obviously remain aware of it. But if it has healed enough for you to have forgotten about it, you can be sure it's not lurking there, waiting to give you an unpleasant surprise. If you suddenly get an unexpected attack of back pain, you shouldn't blame some old, long-ignored accident. The likeliest explanation is the "last straw" syndrome: you have placed an unaccustomed strain on some part of your spine that has been gradually weakened by natural wear and tear.

But let's not make it sound any worse than it is. Although sprains can be very painful, they are rarely permanent, and even the few that persist indefinitely will produce only temporary episodes of pain, not permanent disability. And the symptoms can often be reduced further by simple care and exercise.

What is a torsion injury?

Torsion and torque are terms borrowed from physics, both meaning rotation or, simply, twisting. In its extreme form, it's the most damaging of all back movements.

Then shouldn't extreme twisting be considered just another form of trauma, rather than a separate cause of back pain?

Yes, if the twisting happens to a healthy back. As you remember, that's what was happening to the young weight-lifter I described in Chapter 1, who was twisting his back so violently doing his "home-made" exercises. But for most of us the torsion affects discs that have already begun to dry out and fray a little.

Exactly how does torsion injure my spine?

If you twist your spine hard enough and often enough, some of the radial-ply fibers in the shells of the discs become slack. Gradually the discs lose their normal resistance to rotation. The more you twist, the easier it becomes for you to stretch those fibers still further. If the excessive rotation continues, the fibers will weaken and may eventually tear. This kind of torque shouldn't be confused with a controlled rotation exercise that can strengthen the trunk muscles and actually protect the discs from injury.

The damage can be more extensive if you combine torsion and load; that is, if you twist your back while some extra weight is bearing down on your spine. For example, if you're working in a warehouse where you must twist to lift heavy cartons from a shelf and place them on a conveyor belt. If you do that long enough by rotating the upper part of your body, instead of using your feet to turn around, you are combining torsion and load in a way that can injure your spine.

What actually happens to your spine when, to use your example, you twist your body while lifting that heavy box?

To understand that you need to know a little more spinal anatomy. The outer shell of the disc is not attached directly to the bone of the vertebra. Rather, it is attached by means of a fibrous cartilage plate known as the end plate. The end plate adheres directly to the flat surface of the bone. When your spine is subjected to extreme torsion under load, a small fragment of the end plate can be ripped right off the vertebra, creating a form of Type Two back pain.

What can be done for a person whose back is injured in this way?

Although the problem involves an end-plate rupture, the result is just another form of disc bulge. If the protruding portion of the end plate and disc wall are close to a nerve root we may have Type Three problems. In either case, most of these people will get better with rest and proper exercise. Very few will need surgery.

The damage can also lead to segmental instability, and we have already talked about the treatment for that.

How do you reconcile your description of common backache with the back problems we all hear about, such as "slipped disc," or "herniated disc" or "disintegrating disc" or "degenerative disc disease"?

I don't try to reconcile them. I concentrate instead on trying to get across the message that many terms you hear used to describe back problems are misnomers, and others are just fancy or long-winded terms for conditions that can be described more sensibly in ordinary language. A herniated disc, for instance, is just a ruptured disc that went to college.

Another part of the confusion arises from the fact that there is an indistinct progression from a disc that is mildly bulging to one that is herniated. From physical examination, it's impossible to tell whether the disc has bulged almost to the breaking point or has actually begun to rupture. There are no changes in the Type Two symptoms. As we've already seen, Type Three pain (pressure on a nerve) can result from a disc that merely bulges or from one where the nucleus has begun to escape.

Among the misnomers, "disintegrating disc" is a fraudulent term. Discs may dry out a little with age but they don't disintegrate. The notorious "slipped disc" is the most pervasive and demoralizing misnomer of all. I wish I had a dollar for every time I've had to explain to someone that there is no such thing. The fibrous outer shells of the discs are so firmly embedded in the cartilage of the end plate that they can't possibly slip out of place. Even if you got struck in the back by a speeding bus, the impact could break the vertebrae without dislodging the discs. That's how firmly the discs are positioned.

The "slipped disc" is just one of those figures of speech that persist as folklore. Some doctors use it although they know how inaccurate and misleading it can be. It's not something they readily admit doing, however. Often when I speak to medical audiences I ask for a show of hands to see how many of my listeners use the term "slipped disc" when discussing backs with their patients. Nobody ever raises a hand. Several years ago, while working in an out-patient department, I overheard the orthopedic surgeon in the next cubicle telling his patient that she had a slipped disc. I felt a strong urge to leap into the room and accuse him of being the one who's going around North America spreading all this misunderstanding.

"Degenerative disc disease" is another phrase that invites confusion. Some doctors use the term – mostly, I suspect, because it abbreviates conveniently as "DDD" in the notes they write for patients' files. All that DDD means, really, is wear and tear. I object to the use of a pretentious word like "degenerative" instead of "wearing out," but I am far more upset by the use of the word "disease." By any reasonable definition, wear and tear is not a disease, whether it occurs in a facet joint during the normal use of your spine, or in the palm of your hand during a tug-of-war contest. ("Stop the tug-of-war and call the doctor, Ma! I've got degenerating palm disease!")

I dislike the term not only because it overstates the seriousness of simple aging but also because it's likely to send patients off in search of a cure – and we're not talking about a curable affliction. We're talking about a condition that has to be managed over a long period to prevent avoidable wear and to give nature time to contribute to the healing process.

But surely a lot of terms we hear aren't just folklore or fancy phrases. Arthritis, for instance – isn't it a disease that often attacks the spine?

No, arthritis is not a disease, either. It's just a description meaning "inflamed joint." It says nothing about why the inflammation has occurred. And, as you no doubt realize, a joint can become inflamed for many different reasons.

Let's assume that I am hurrying out of a room and I accidentally slam the door on my thumb. Immediately the joint of my thumb becomes swollen and sore. Does that make me an arthritis sufferer? Most people would say no, but the correct answer is yes. Technically, any time one or more of my joints are inflamed I have arthritis.

The term arthritis, then, doesn't convey much useful meaning unless it's accompanied by an adjective or phrase indicating what caused it. The type of arthritis that comes from injuring a joint is called traumatic arthritis. The inflammation that develops in the facet joints of the spine as a result of the natural wear and tear of aging is called osteoarthritis. And, as you might suppose, the word "arthritis" is used with various other adjectives to denote joint inflammation from various other causes.

For that reason, you can't expect to get a helpful answer if you go to your doctor and say, "I've got arthritis – what should I do about it?" All you are telling him, at the very most, is that you have an inflamed joint, or, more likely, just that you have a sore joint. Without knowing *why* the joint is sore, the doctor has no information on which to prescribe treatment. He must determine the cause of your arthritis before he can help you.

But doesn't the arthritis society run ads on television and in the newspapers suggesting that arthritis is a terrible disease for which they are trying to find a cure?

That's right. I remember one of their TV commercials. It showed people's hands with the joints grotesquely deformed by rheumatoid disease. But the message was: "Beware of arthritis."

Isn't that a form of misleading advertising?

Yes, but I suppose they would argue that all they have done is leave out the qualifying adjective to keep the message clear and simple, since the public really doesn't care whether they are seeing rheumatoid arthritis, osteoarthritis, traumatic arthritis, or any other kind, for that matter. After all, a commercial is supposed to be an attention-getter, not a scientific lesson. And it *is* all in a good cause, since the society is trying to find a way to prevent or cure diseases that cause joints to become inflamed. Nobody can quarrel with an aim like that, but the unfortunate side effect is that the word arthritis becomes impressed in many people's minds as the name of a serious disease instead of what it is – merely a description of an inflamed joint.

Matters are only made worse by the fact that many doctors use the word casually and incorrectly to describe a wide range of conditions that can produce sore joints – the well-known "touch of arthritis."

In fact, the notion of arthritis as a disease is so thoroughly entrenched in our thinking that some back patients refuse to believe that their inflamed joints are the result of nothing more than wear and tear. In their view, wear and tear may be something that happens to other patients' backs, but their own problem is the "disease" they know as arthritis. And that's a shame, because as long as they see their condition that way, they are unlikely to be interested in the simple preventive measures that can help them.

Then you're not objecting just because some people don't use certain words according to the definitions in some medical dictionary.

Certainly not. I object in general to the misuse of a word like arthritis for two very practical reasons. First, because the misused word often displaces a term that could tell you something useful; and, second, because it often conveys a false impression in a patient's mind. A patient will ask me, "If I have arthritis in my shoulder, will it spread to my spine?" Obviously, the person is thinking of arthritis as a disease capable of moving around the body, wreaking pain and destruction wherever it goes. But now that you understand what arthritis really means, you can see that although the concern is valid, the question is meaningless. Any possible spread depends on the underlying cause of the problem and not on the mere presence of an inflamed joint.

I am just as critical, by the way, when medical people confuse their patients by speaking the language of Doctor – deliberately ignoring perfectly useful everyday words in favor of pretentious medical terms. A physician addicted to speaking Doctor may tell a patient, for instance, that he has "a myofascial sprain" when he could simply say "a pulled muscle."

I'm beginning to suspect that Doctor as a language is even more contagious than many of the afflictions it describes. I was sitting down for a haircut the other day when my barber suddenly announced that I had *alopecia areata*. The very idea would have paralyzed me with fright if I hadn't happened to know that *alopecia areata*, in simple English, is a bald spot. And in fact it wasn't even *that* – it was only a cut from a minor mishap several weeks earlier. I should have countered him by saying he'd been standing around in his shop so long that he'd developed a bad case of *pes planus* – that's Doctor for flat feet.

Some technical terms are necessary, of course, because they have no equivalents in ordinary language. But many terms you hear add little, and doctors would be performing a great service by abandoning them when they're talking to their patients.

How can a patient tell, then, which terms are significant and which are just fancy ways of saying ordinary things?

Any time your doctor uses a term you don't understand, ask what it means. Never be ashamed to admit you don't know some medical word or phrase. Medical people don't know them all either, and many of them speak poor Doctor.

The word sciatica is a good example. Sciatica means acute leg pain caused by direct pressure on a nerve. But by sloppy usage it has come to mean any leg pain associated with back trouble. And, as I have mentioned, leg pain is a symptom of all four types of common backache, whereas only Type Three produces true sciatica. And so if I merely tell another doctor that a patient has sciatica I may be using the word correctly, but the other doctor can easily misunderstand the meaning.

We've talked a lot about common backache, but there must be specific diseases that cause pain in the back.

Yes, and there are two in particular that ought to be mentioned here. One is ankylosing spondylitis; the other is rheumatoid disease.

Ankylosing spondylitis is primarily a young man's disease, with very distinctive characteristics. These include a visible flattening of the surface of the low back, loss of chest movement, progressive stiffness in the joints of the spine, and, in about half of all cases, stiffness in the hips or knees. The spinal stiffness is particularly noticeable first thing in the morning, and it is greatly relieved by exercise or almost any form of physical activity. If you think I have just described your symptoms, ask your doctor for an examination. There are some X-rays and blood tests which can rule out this and several other diseases that affect the back.

Rheumatoid disease is a condition in which the body reacts against itself, behaving as though it were coping with a foreign substance. It's a process that can affect many parts of the body including the nervous system, the internal organs, the skin, and, of course, the joints. If the joints are affected they become inflamed and eventually damaged. This aspect of the disease is called rheumatoid arthritis.

Obviously, it can be a serious affliction at its worst, but the great majority of patients with rheumatoid disease do very well. And to keep it in perspective: only 2 percent of the population have the disease, and only 10 percent of *those* people have severe joint problems. What those percentages mean, then, is that only two people out of a thousand suffer severe joint problems from rheumatoid arthritis. In contrast, about 800 out of every thousand people, at some time in their lives, suffer from common backache.

Then only a tiny fraction of all back pain sufferers have arthritis caused by rheumatoid disease?

Exactly. But can you imagine how many of them saw that TV commercial depicting rheumatoid arthritis – and how upset and frightened they would have been if their doctors told them later that they had a "touch of arthritis" in their spines?

Yet we know from statistics that most of those people have nothing more than a minor case of Type One or Type Two back pain. Their backs are hurting simply because the facet joints are worn. That's the extent of their arthritis.

Then you're not just quibbling when you insist on correct usage of terms like arthritis.

Far from it. A talented writer once said, "The difference between the *right* word and the *almost-right* word is like the difference between a lightning bolt and a lightning bug."

As a back patient, do yourself a favor: don't be frightened by words. Those lightning bolts you're worrying about may well turn out to be nothing more than lightning bugs.

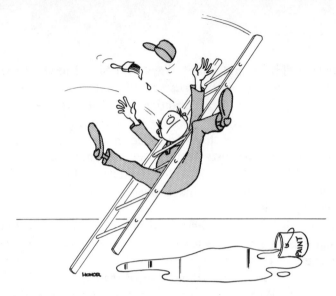

4. "WHIPLASH" AND OTHER FOLKLORE

As an author, lecturer, and physician, I have seldom passed up an opportunity to poke fun at the idea of the "slipped disc." It's one of the great fallacies of our time, and I like to think my efforts have helped reduce popular belief in this frightening and erroneous phrase. Unfortunately, it's only one of several common and misleading expressions that create a lot of unnecessary apprehension and fear.

This chapter is devoted to three such misunderstood terms. One is that special favorite of the legal profession: whiplash.

The other two are the broken neck and the broken back. Both are injuries that can, of course, be extremely serious. But, contrary to popular impression, they do not automatically consign their victims to paralysis or death. Right at this moment there are people walking around with broken backs who'll tell you they have nothing ailing them but a few stiff muscles. And I've seen many patients with broken necks who have recovered and now have no neck pain at all.

Is it true that whiplash is one of the most serious ailments you can have?

You have just expressed a basic misconception shared by many people. However, *whiplash is not an ailment or physical injury at all but an action* that occurs to the neck under certain specific conditions and may or may not cause injury.

The commonest situation, as you probably know, is a traffic accident where the victim is riding in a car that is struck from the rear. Being rear-ended by another car is not the same as being in the car that does the rear-ending. They involve two entirely different forms of impact, and they propel you in distinctly different ways.

If you are in a high-speed accident where your car rear-ends another vehicle or crashes into some other obstacle, your body may be restrained but your head is thrown forward. It can't bob forward very far before your chin hits your chest. That may hurt a lot. It may bruise your chin and wrench your back muscles. But the action is limited, and because your neck is protected from further movement, there is no whiplash effect.

Now consider what happens if you're in the car that gets rear-ended in a high-speed collision. Let's assume your car seat is not equipped with a head-rest. When the vehicle behind you smashes into your car, your whole body, from the shoulders down, is suddenly propelled forward. Your head, having nothing in back of it, gets left behind. In this situation, there is no equivalent of your chin striking your chest, and so your head snaps backward as far as it can go. (Some victims recall having their heads thrown back so far that for a split second they actually caught an upside-down glimpse of the car's rear window.) An instant after this violent backward motion, your head recoils forward with almost equal force.

Your neck, which lacks the protective structure of your middle and lower spine, has just been subjected to whiplash. And, of course, the more violently your head is thrown backward and forward in that lashing motion, the greater the strain on the muscles, ligaments, and joints in your neck. That's why a rear-end collision poses a greater threat to your neck than colliding head-on.

Is it true that once you've suffered from whiplash your neck will never be normal again?

That depends on the nature and extent of the injury. If it's really severe, the ligaments that stabilize the bones in your neck could be torn, some joints in your upper spine could be severely sprained, or several vertebrae could be fractured. But if you're in a low-speed rear-end collision where that whiplashing action is minimal, you may sustain only minor injuries or no injuries at all.

I'm beginning to see why you say whiplash is not actually an ailment or physical injury.

It's one of those words that confuses an issue. Although you may *experience* whiplash, there is no such thing as *having* whiplash in the sense of having a sore joint or a sprained ligament in your neck. Whiplash, in other words, is just a way of getting hurt. There are lots of ways to get hurt, as we all know. You can slip on an icy sidewalk or walk into a brick wall or fall off a ladder.

If I called you up on the phone and told you I fell off a ladder last weekend, you'd wonder whether I merely skinned a knee or was lying in a hospital with two broken legs and several cracked ribs. You'd ask, "Were you badly hurt?" You wouldn't say, "Oh, what a terrible thing! You've got ladderfall! My Uncle George, the house painter, got ladderfall once, and he almost died!"

Yet people talk that way about whiplash, not realizing that, like "ladderfall," it's a term that describes a possibly injurious action but says nothing about the actual damage – if any. That's why it's meaningless to say, "I've got whiplash – will I ever be normal again?" Or, "What's the treatment for whiplash?" The answers depend on what injuries occurred and how serious they are.

You may be technically right, but my sister's doctor told her she had whiplash – and her lawyer even proved it in court.

That doesn't surprise me. Lawyers misuse the term all the time, and so do some doctors. A woman who had been in a car accident years earlier came to see me about neck pain. In the course of relating her medical background, she made a point of repeating something she was told right after the accident. A young doctor (fresh out of medical school, I suspect) examined her neck and announced that she had the worst case of whiplash he had ever seen.

Never mind that probably this young doctor had never before examined a patient with acute neck pain. Since he was not present at the accident he could not have *seen* her whiplash – only its result. Yet a frightening comment like that, especially from a medical person, can seriously inhibit recovery. This woman honestly believed she had "the worst case of whiplash" in the annals of medicine. There was nothing I could say to convince her she would some day get well.

In contrast to that young doctor, others go to the opposite extreme. Instead of simply rejecting whiplash as a diagnosis and explaining that it's a mechanical action, some doctors deny that there's any such thing at all. And so the patient hears that opinion from the doctor, only to hear it contradicted by his lawyer, who probably sees "whiplash" as a magic word worth several thousand dollars in court. And, of course, when it suits their argument in litigation, lawyers can make a whiplash injury sound far worse than it is.

Lawyers also apply the term far too broadly, sometimes using it to mean a neck injury of any kind. Obviously, they savor the sound of the word. I have to admit "whiplash" sounds a lot more dramatic and damaging than "sprain" or even "torn ligament." Unfortunately, there are some doctors who do not hesitate to use the term when testifying in court. It's not hard to guess which witness the jury would find more convincing – the specialist who details the horrors of whiplash or the one who drones on about minor soft-tissue injury.

Some lawyers codify this misconception further by putting price tags on this non-existent diagnosis. I've heard them talk about a client having "a five-thousand-dollar whipper" ("whipper" being Lawyer for a whiplash injury). In this example, five thousand dollars does not refer, as you might assume, to the patient's medical costs. It's the amount the lawyer calculates the "whiplash" might generate in settling a court case. And I can hardly blame anyone for reasoning that if whiplash is worth that kind of money in a court of law, it must surely be a real and serious condition.

Do head-rests on car seats help prevent the whiplash effect?

The good ones do, but most head-rests are poorly designed or incorrectly positioned. They are almost always too low. A head-rest is useless behind your neck. To provide the support needed to prevent the whiplash action, it must be behind your head.

I suggest that all car owners check their head-rests to see that they're high enough. If a head-rest is too low and cannot be adjusted, it should be replaced. That may be costly, but it will be well worth the money if it can prevent a serious neck injury. In certain circumstances, a properly installed head-rest can prove as important to safety as a seat belt. And while we're on the subject, I can testify from professional experience that seat belts save lives and prevent many serious injuries, and I urge every driver and passenger to use them.

You've explained what whiplash is but you haven't said much about the injuries it can cause. Can whiplash break a person's neck?

Yes – although, as I said earlier, a broken neck is not necessarily fatal or crippling. When your head is whiplashed back and forth, the ligament along the front of the spinal column may be torn. If it tears loose, it may take with it a little bit of bone from the front of a vertebra. And, technically, that's a broken neck – a fracture in this case caused by whiplash. (I never use those terms without reminding people that there is no difference between a break and a fracture or a crack. They all mean the same thing.)

People worry a lot about broken necks and broken backs, and I don't blame them. According to popular mythology, a broken back will paralyze you for life and a broken neck will kill you. These notions are not entirely fictional, of course. They're based on true stories of very serious mishaps – people diving into shallow pools or getting their necks snapped in skiing accidents. But for every life-threatening case there are hundreds of cases of broken vertebrae that are almost inconsequential.

I've seen patients who had broken necks and didn't even know it. And yet in each instance the break was there to be seen by X-ray. The person didn't realize it was a fracture because it hurt no more than a muscle spasm would. Perhaps the break occurred because bone had grown abnormally thin, as it does with the osteoporosis found in older people. In such cases, the only symptom may be a bit of temporary neck pain.

It must be touchy to tell a patient, "You've got a broken neck."

In cases like that, I'm very careful about what I say – or, more precisely, how I say it. I want people to realize that a broken neck is not necessarily a serious problem. And, knowing what the typical view is, I'm wary of causing needless alarm. Unless the question comes up directly, I tend not to use the term "broken neck." Instead, I would describe the problem in more specific terms, by saying something like, "There's a small crack in one vertebra. . ."

I gather that even when it is very painful, a broken neck is unlikely to be life-threatening.

Yes, that's true. One good example is an injury known as clay shoveler's fracture, which occurs in the lowest of the seven vertebrae in your neck. That's the bone that forms a little bump at the point where, so to speak, your neck joins your back.

Clay shoveler's fracture is exactly what it sounds like: an injury that occurs when someone digs into clay or other hard ground. He stabs the point of the shovel into the soil but it doesn't give. The shovel stops dead, sending a jolt up through the person's arms and shoulders. His back muscles react with such tension that they tear away a wing-like part of the vertebra called the "spinous process."

I know that sounds horrible, and certainly it's painful, but it's not as damaging as you might suppose. It doesn't affect the function of the neck or the nerves. It's a broken neck in the true sense of the term but it has no serious consequences.

How do you treat a clay shoveler's fracture?

There's no need to treat it. The spinous process heals by itself. The victim is in pain and won't feel like using a shovel for a few months. But otherwise he is okay.

My main point is that there are many forms of broken necks and broken backs that you don't often hear about because they aren't dramatic or dangerous.

Let's talk about the serious cases.

All right, but they, too, need to be kept in perspective. A broken neck can be very serious. If a bone in your neck is fractured and dislocated, it may move and cut the spinal cord. And if that cut occurs above the level of the nerves that control the diaphragm, you stop breathing and die.

But the human body can survive some devastating injuries and eventually mend itself. I had one patient who suffered a broken neck in a car accident. The car ran off the road into a deep ditch, rolling over several times. The man doesn't know exactly what happened but he remembers having to lift his head by his hair; he couldn't raise it any other way. He had broken the vertebra near the top of the neck that permits the head to rotate from side to side. The broken bone had shifted slightly out of place, but luckily there was no damage to the spinal cord, and his nervous system was functioning normally.

For treatment, he was fitted with an outfit called a halo vest, which is now standard equipment for such cases. The halo is fastened to the skull with specially designed screws, and mounted on metal posts, which are attached to a shoulder harness and incorporated into a plastic vest. The idea, of course, is to immobilize the neck until it mends.

This fellow wore that outfit for about four months. He wasn't comfortable but he was up and around. Certainly it was better than the old-style treatment, which would have kept him flat on a turning frame for the same time, in traction provided by a pair of skull tongs.

After the prescribed time, the halo vest was removed. The fracture had healed, and the man's neck was normal again. I mention this case not because the recovery was exceptional – it wasn't – but because the outcome is typical of what patients with this sort of serious injury can expect.

You did say earlier, though, that the neck lacks the protective structure of the middle and lower spine. Does that mean my neck is more vulnerable than my back?

Yes, it is. Your neck contains seven vertebrae interspersed with discs. These are the cervical vertebrae, and they are designated (from the top down) as C_1 through C_7. The C_1 is called the atlas, named for the Titan from Greek mythology who bore the earth on his back and the heavens on his shoulders.

The atlas is unlike any other vertebra in your spine. A ring-shaped bone with flat surfaces, top and bottom, it balances two small prominences extending from the base of the skull. The atlas is joined to the second (or C_2) vertebra, called the axis, which has a peg known as the "odontoid process" that sticks up through the front of the C_1 ring and is held in place by very strong ligaments. This peg-in-a-hole arrangement permits you to rotate your head from side to side. (The odontoid was the part that got broken in the case of the car accident victim I mentioned; you can understand why he had trouble lifting or turning his head.)

Passing down behind that "tooth" is the spinal cord, which comes out of a hole in the skull, passes through the ring of C_1 and through the hole behind the odontoid process of C_2.

The other five neck bones (C_3 through C_7) are much like the vertebrae in the lower back, except that they are smaller, and the holes forming the spinal canal, for the spinal cord, are proportionately larger.

The facet joints in the neck, instead of being L-shaped like those in the low back, are flat, like clutch plates in a car. Because of their shape, your neck vertebrae don't interlock the way the vertebrae do in your lumbar spine. They rely instead on joint capsules and ligaments to hold them in place.

Like any movable joint, a facet joint can be dislocated. Dislocation is the complete separation of one joint surface from another. Because of their structure, neck joints are more likely to be dislocated than low back joints. In the low back, you'll never find a dislocation unless one or more bones are broken. In your neck, it's possible to have a dislocation without a fracture.

I gather that cases of broken backs run the same gamut as broken necks, from minor to serious.

Yes, they do. As you can appreciate by now, the concept of the broken back is far too broad and vague to have any real meaning. We think of broken backs as occurring in horrendous traffic collisions or falls from tall buildings. These injuries do occur, of course, and can be fatal or leave permanent and serious disability. But a broken back can be the result of something as mild and simple as a sneeze in the case of a person with osteoporosis. The sneeze – or, more precisely, the pressure that a sneeze exerts on the spine – can crush a vertebra slightly, and that, technically, is a broken back. If you break your back that way, you will suffer some pain for about six weeks but there will be no serious results – no instability of your spine, no nerve damage, no degenerative change. The bone will heal by itself, and you may not even realize it was crushed.

In another situation, you can have an injury to the vertebrae when the back muscles suddenly tense up and pull off one of the "transverse processes," which are other wing-like projections on the sides of the vertebrae. Or if you get hit in the back hard enough, those little wings may crack. In either case, you have a broken back.

But, again, these are not serious injuries. Usually, the breaks heal quickly and easily, the muscles reattach themselves, and you are soon feeling fine. Nothing important will have changed – not the structure, the stability, the nerve function, or anything else. Even when a detached transverse process fails to mend itself, it remains captive within its assembly of muscles and ligaments and presents no serious problem. Mind you, it will be painful from the outset – a broken bone always is – and the pain may last for months. But hurt, as I have pointed out before, is not the same as harm.

Then you never consider performing surgery after a break of that kind?

No. In fact, most people who break their backs do not require surgery. The back has a tremendous ability for recovery and a great margin of protection. I already mentioned crushed vertebrae. You may find this hard to believe, but in a serious accident it's possible for a vertebra to be crushed – usually at the front – until it is only two-thirds of its normal height, and yet the victim will suffer only temporary pain. The body gradually adjusts to the new situation.

An older person with osteoporosis may end up with half a dozen or more crushed vertebrae over a period of years. The condition is easy to spot: the crushed vertebrae, being wedge-shaped instead of uniform height front and back, give the spine an unnatural forward curve, making the person round-shouldered.

In appearance, it's quite a pronounced abnormality and can lead to chronic backache, but it causes no nerve damage or other problems. And so, spinal fracture, per se, doesn't call for surgery.

There must be some cases when surgery *is* called for?

Yes. For example, surgery is advisable when a vertebra is not just crushed but shattered. This is what we call a burst fracture, and it is dangerous because fragments of bone can become lodged in the spinal canal, where they may interfere with the nervous system and cause partial paralysis.

Until a few years ago, this condition was hard to diagnose, because the injury cannot be seen with any certainty on conventional X-ray or even on a myelogram. Now, thanks to the computerized axial tomograph scanner – the diagnostic machine usually known simply as the CT or CAT scan – we can identify these "bursts" of the bone quite precisely. Once they have been located, a surgeon can go in and remove them. Incidentally, this is usually done from the front of the patient's body, because that route normally provides better access to the fracture fragments.

After that operation will a paralyzed person usually regain his or her normal functions?

The amount of paralysis will depend largely on the damage done to the spinal cord or to the *cauda equina* at the time of injury. But, obviously, if pressure from the bone fragments continues, removing these fragments gives the patient the best possible chance for recovery. Unfortunately, unlike so many other parts of the body, the spinal cord has very limited powers of regeneration, and once serious damage has occurred there may be little chance for a return of normal function.

My main point, however, is that while surgery is called for when there is a specific task to perform, such as restoring adequate stability or removing bone fragments from the spinal canal, most vertebral injuries can be safely left to heal by themselves. And that includes a good many broken backs.

One example is the Chance fracture, which was first described back in the 1940s by a doctor with the delightfully unlikely name of Quigley Chance.

Chance fractures are hardly ever seen any more. They were more common some years ago, when most cars had lap-type seat belts, with no shoulder restraints. When a passenger is involved in a violent, head-on collision while wearing a lap belt, the belly has no time to compress. The person's body is folded over the belt, with all the bending taking place at the front of the abdomen. This abnormal bending pattern can literally tear the spine apart. The discs in the spine are so tough and so securely attached that they are not affected, but the bone, being weaker, is torn in two. In an X-ray it looks as though someone has taken a cheese cutter and sliced the bone in half and then yanked the two pieces apart, creating a gap that may be a quarter of an inch wide.

Are you saying that people can survive such a horrible injury?

Yes – although you wouldn't think so if you could read the X-ray. And yet, usually after a few months he or she will be walking around with no serious nerve damage whatever and certainly with no paralysis. Typically, the only complaint is back pain, which gradually subsides as the gap between the two pieces of the vertebra eventually fills up with new bone growth so that the spine functions normally.

You've certainly convinced me that whiplash and broken necks and backs are not necessarily the life-shattering experiences that most people suppose.

I hope I have. I don't want to minimize the seriousness of the injuries that occur in some cases, but it's important to keep things in perspective. Otherwise, some people will worry needlessly about life-long disabilities arising out of accidents from which, in reality, they will recover nicely.

Sometimes people have anxieties about complications that can't possibly happen. For instance, I've talked to patients and their relatives who were afraid that a person who has been injured in the low back might have damaged the spinal cord. Happily, I can dispel that fear by pointing out one simple fact: in that lowest part of your spine, there *is* no spinal cord, only a bundle of more resilient nerve roots.

Surely you don't expect people to be walking around with that kind of medical information in their heads.

No, of course not. I expect people to spend their time thinking about matters of more immediate concern than how their bodies work or what certain medical and pseudo-medical terms mean. But I do hope that readers who find themselves in emergency wards, either as accident victims or as attending relatives, will be able to remember the information in this chapter and keep things in perspective.

If anyone tells you someone "has whiplash," or is suffering from "a broken neck" or "a broken back," I hope you'll realize that the situation is probably not nearly as bad as it sounds. Your best response is to ask exactly what the damage is and what the consequences are likely to be.

Ninety-nine times out of a hundred, if you ignore those ominous phrases and all the emotional baggage that goes with them, you can draw a lot of comfort from learning the facts and remembering how adept the human body is at surviving injury and healing itself.

5. ABOUT THAT PAIN IN YOUR NECK

Like many people, I'm seldom satisfied with my first attempt at anything, and I tend to worry long after it's too late to make changes. Whether it's a matter of planning an "ideal" house, or writing a first book, most of us look back on the finished product and see things we wish we'd done differently.

In the case of my first book, *The Back Doctor*, I didn't have to do the second-guessing alone; my readers offered me numerous comments that proved most helpful when the time came to plan this second volume. Many of them told me they wished I had said more about neck pain. Originally I thought I had covered the subject thoroughly enough in a book which, after all, was written primarily for people with bad backs. Even at that, the index lists sixteen references under "neck" and four others under "cervical spine."

Necks and low backs, of course, have many problems in common. They are, after all, both parts of the same biomechanical system. But many of the specific questions I was asked about the nature and treatment of neck pain were not answered in my first book.

This chapter, then, is intended to deal with the concerns I have heard expressed so often in the past half-dozen years. Certainly I have never underestimated the importance of neck pain. A full

50 percent of all the people who come to me with back problems have neck pain as well, and some 20 to 30 percent of all my patients are people with nothing *but* neck pain.

And so I dedicate this chapter to those two groups and others like them for whom neck pain is, or might become, a problem.

My doctor keeps referring to my problem as neck pain, and yet the pain really isn't in my neck. The worst of it is along the top of my shoulder and beside my shoulder blade.

If your pain runs along the inner border of your shoulder blade, it probably comes from your neck. I understand why you might think there is something wrong with your shoulder, because that's where it hurts. But often that's not where the trouble originates.

It can be quite confusing. I have a simple test I use to separate pain referred from the neck from pain arising in the shoulder itself, and it's something you can try for yourself:

Place one hand over the most painful area. Now take careful note of the location. If your hand is over the upper part of the arm, you probably have true shoulder pain. But if your hand is on top of your shoulder, it is more likely you have neck pain that is radiating into the area.

Are you saying all neck pain is felt on top of the shoulder?

By no means. Commonly, neck pain is literally, as well as figuratively, a pain in the neck. Usually you'll feel the pain most intensely in the back of your neck, and often that's because the muscles there are in spasm. Sometimes the pain radiates downward into your shoulders and back because the spasm spreads into the *trapezius*, a big kite-shaped muscle that starts with a point at the base of your skull, reaches the tips of both shoulders, and extends down over much of your back to another point on your spine above the waist.

When spasms occur, you are likely to notice little tight knots along the upper ridge of *trapezius* muscle on top of your shoulders.

This is a location where emotional tension is often felt. And if it is your neck pain that is making you tense, you get a double whammy: pain from the original cause, plus pain from the muscular tension.

Of course it's possible to have neck and shoulder pain at the same time from separate causes. In fact 10 to 20 percent of all people with neck pain have separate (though usually related) trouble in the shoulder. Your shoulders are contained in rather loose capsules that permit a wide range of movement, but if the joints are kept immobile – as they often are when neck pain spreads to the shoulder area – the folds of that capsule get stuck together. Soon you find you can't raise your arm without pain, and every attempt to move the shoulder increases the agony. The area around the joint is bound with scar tissue, and every time you move you tear it a little. This condition is aptly described as "frozen shoulder."

The same thing can happen to your shoulder if you break your wrist. Putting your wrist in a cast and your arm in a sling immobilizes the shoulder. To avoid the risk of having your shoulder seize up, you shouldn't wear the sling any longer than a couple of weeks. For the same reason, the therapy for a person recovering from a broken wrist will routinely include practicing shoulder movement.

A friend of mine told me she had pain that apparently started in her neck and went past her shoulders all the way down her arms into her hands. Is this possible?

Yes, that can certainly happen. More often, there is pain radiating into the shoulder and upper arm, about as far as the elbow, with tingling, numbing, or burning sensations down into the hand.

The fact that the symptoms are felt in areas other than the neck doesn't mean the pain is any less intense. The pain you mentioned that radiates from your neck down along your shoulder blades can be especially troublesome. In fact, it can become the dominant problem – deep-seated, sometimes causing nausea, and usually aggravated by any sort of movement or the slightest tensing of the muscles. Often, it's not even relieved by lying down and trying to relax. That pain can be excruciating, as I know from personal experience.

As you may realize, the process of pain radiating from the neck is much the same as the pain that spreads into the legs when someone has low-back trouble. In that case, the worst pain is often in the thighs, hips, or buttocks.

This similarly won't surprise you if you understand something of the structure of the human nervous system. In your neck, six nerve roots on each side combine into an elaborate arrangement called the *brachial plexus*, which sends three major nerves into your arm to perform specific functions. In your low back, you have a comparable group of nerve roots, which join together to form the more familiar sciatic nerve. It's actually a bundle of nerves that run down the leg to perform specific functions there.

As a result, if a certain nerve root leaving your spine detects a painful condition in the back, you may feel symptoms in the distant location which that nerve supplies. This spread is called referred pain and must be differentiated from pain running into the arm or leg because of actual nerve damage. One nerve commonly involved with referred pain exits between the fifth and sixth vertebrae in your neck and runs down to your thumb and forefinger. (In anatomical terms, there are seven cervical vertebrae numbered from the top. This nerve appears between cervical five and cervical six, or C_5-C_6.)

To describe the condition from the diagnostician's point of view, if you told me you felt pain or unpleasant sensations in your thumb and forefinger, I'd suspect your trouble was originating at the C_5-C_6 level, in the lower part of your neck.

You seem to be saying that pain originating in your spine is much the same whether it's in your neck or down in your low back.

Broadly speaking, that's true. The pain-producing mechanisms are similar; both your neck and your back can experience pain from wear and tear in the facet joints and discs – Type One and Type Two pain, in other words. But with Type Three pain, a pinched nerve, it's usually a different story. As we saw in Chapter 3, when a nerve in the low back is pinched, the problem is caused by either a bulging or ruptured disc or a bony entrapment. If you have neck pain from a pinched nerve, however, the culprit is likely a combination of pressure from the bone and disc.

Incidentally, one other difference worth noting here is another basic point of anatomy: as we discussed in Chapter 4, your neck is built for more mobility than your low back. That means as the years go by and your discs dry out and your spinal joints lose some of their flexibility, you'll notice the change more in your neck than in your back, simply because you expect your neck to be more flexible. You can see that difference if you watch someone back a car out of a driveway. A young adult at the wheel will simply turn the head around as far as necessary to see out the back window. But a driver who is, say, fifty or older will have to turn the whole upper body to get the necessary view.

It seems to me that many of the people I've known with stiff, painful necks also had frequent headaches. Is that also a matter of referred pain?

In some cases it is. But whether it's referred pain or muscle tension pain doesn't make a lot of immediate difference. In fact, the two are so closely associated that they are almost indistinguishable. Neck pain is usually felt through spasm in half a dozen small neck muscles that relate to head and neck movement, and these muscles are part of a larger muscle mass covering the entire skull. When the little muscles are irritated, the muscles overlying the skull become tense, and you get a headache. That kind of muscle tension is by far the commonest cause of all headaches, whether or not they are accompanied or triggered by neck pain.

Is a muscle-tension headache the same as a migraine?

Definitely not. Migraine is a term that is often misused. Many of my neck pain patients mistakenly describe their headaches as migraines. To them, the word just means severe. A true migraine is caused by alterations in the function of the cranial blood vessels. The symptoms of the common or the classic migraine can vary a great deal, but typically the pain is one-sided (although bilateral headaches are not rare) and accompanied by a loss of appetite, nausea, and sometimes vomiting. Often before the headache starts there is a period when the victim feels inappropriate mood swings or sudden cravings. In the classic migraine there is a period of visual disturbances, an "aura." A migraine attack can wake a sufferer from a sound sleep, something a muscle-tension headache won't do. One fact that surprises many of my patients is that the migraine headache doesn't always produce excruciating pain.

Muscle-tension headaches begin insidiously and disappear slowly and haltingly. The pain can last for days, far longer than the normal migraine. The associated nausea is usually caused by a misuse of pain medication.

My main point, though, is that "migraine" refers to a specific condition which can be accurately diagnosed, and should not be used to denote just any sort of severe headache, regardless of its nature or cause.

Are psychological factors important in neck pain?

They certainly are. It's no mere coincidence that a worrisome situation is often described as a pain in the neck; worry or anxiety can easily trigger neck pain by increasing muscle tension. Once the muscle spasm starts, you are in danger of falling into one of those loops where pain causes suffering, suffering causes tension, and tension completes the loop by increasing the pain.

Earlier, you described how neck pain can be carried by the nerves down into the arms and even into the fingers. Does that indicate that a nerve is damaged? Does it mean I have a pinched nerve?

To answer your second question first: nerve damage is not the same thing as a pinched nerve. A nerve may be squeezed and become painful without being damaged. And in answer to your first question: the fact that a pain sensation is being transmitted by a particular nerve – say, from a worn facet joint in the neck down to the elbow – is not necessarily an indication that the nerve itself is in trouble. Chances are the nerve is just doing its job as the messenger, carrying the pain signal without being part of the problem. This is what we mean by referred pain. Blaming the nerve would be like shooting a messenger for bringing you bad news.

Once, when I went to my doctor with neck pain, he told me it was caused by muscle strain. Does that sound plausible to you?

That's perfectly plausible, and he was probably right. Neck pain may be caused either by emotional tension or physical strain. We are vulnerable to the physical strain partly because of the way the human neck is constructed, but mainly because of the demands we make on our necks.

Just as you should if you were suffering from low-back pain, you must make the distinction between hurt and harm. Muscle spasm can be very painful, but it is usually quite harmless. Sitting in a cold draft from an air-conditioner, for example, can cause the neck muscles to tighten and cause pain. If you have simple Type One problems, that extra muscular tension may be enough to irritate the worn joints and increase the discomfort or even produce a typical attack. But unless you understand what is happening, it will seem as if the cold air blew right into your neck and froze it stiff.

The same type of muscle spasm can occur if you sleep in an uncomfortable position or with a pillow that's too thick or springy. Even turning your head suddenly may trigger a painful episode. But, as difficult as the idea may be to accept, in each case the strain and the spasm are harmless.

What can I do to reduce those strains and avoid neck pain?

There are a great many things you can do, and I'll list some of them for you. Not every suggestion will apply to everyone, of course, but I think there's something here for most people who suffer neck pain. And, for that matter, a lot of this advice also applies to people with backache.

 • Make sure your body and your mind are both getting enough rest. That means reasonable intervals of relaxation during your waking day and enough sleep at night. To respect your neck's natural limitations, give it a rest every so often. Whatever you happen to be doing, don't stand or sit in the same position, hour after hour, without a change. Break away every so often, either to rest or to switch to some other activity where those tired neck muscles will have a chance to take it easy. Or, better still, if you're engaged in any activity where the choice is entirely yours, pack it up for a while at the first sign of neck pain.

We all admire achievement, but it's a fact that many people with the worst cases of neck pain are the over-achievers – people who habitually drive themselves beyond the limits of their endurance. Such people, in my view, pay an unnecessarily heavy price for what they accomplish, when a little rest and relaxation could do them so much good. I think they'd achieve just as much that way – more, actually, because they would also succeed in avoiding neck pain.

• Examine your personal relationships. Do they create anger and hostility you can't release? If so, start looking for a harmless way to work off that tension. Physical activity would help – regular workouts in a gym or chopping a little firewood.

• If you're always dashing here and there, habitually late for appointments and obliged to apologize for your tardiness, find ways to reorganize your daily routine. There are good books on time management.

• Consider the possibility that you are working longer and harder than you need to, especially if you are holding down two jobs. Many women are in that situation today, with a household to run and a family to raise as well as a full-time job outside the home. If that's what you're coping with, it may be time for a reassignment of household responsibilities and chores. It isn't easy for some people to give up that responsibility and begin to rely on others. But it may be a choice between keeping your independence or overcoming your neck pain.

• Another enemy is boredom. Spending day after day at the same monotonous routine gives you an unneeded opportunity to dwell on aches and pains not only in your neck or back but also in many other parts of the body. Without a diversion, you may even begin to feel stress from the monotony. If there is no way of adding interest to the job itself, try to find some outside interests during work breaks or after hours.

• Don't overlook the possibility that some physical or emotional injury in the past may be an underlying cause of your muscle tension and pain. Physical irritation can come from sensitive scar tissue at the muscles' attachments to the vertebrae or from an old injury to the facet joints. But, remember, pain from those sorts of problems would have recurred periodically over the years. Once a physical injury to the neck heals painlessly, it isn't likely to start up again. Emotional stress, however, can last long after all the structural problems are resolved. That second possibility is especially strong if you have had to tell yourself to "keep your chin up" – a posture that is all too symbolic of the unnecessary strain we sometimes impose on our necks. Your symptoms may include frequent feelings of sadness and discouragement and a tendency to cry easily.

• Try to avoid dozing off while seated, as so many of us do while watching TV. Napping in an upright position places a great deal of strain on your neck as you allow your head to tip forward, with your chin on your chest. If you feel the need for a nap, go and lie down.

• The way you stand and walk can make a difference. If you slouch around like a high-fashion model, you may develop too much lordosis, or swayback, in your lower spine. This posture will inevitably thrust your head and neck forward and produce unnecessary stress on the muscles and ligaments along your spine.

• Driving a car can cause a lot of neck strain unless you take special steps to avoid it. For one thing, the very act of operating a car in heavy traffic or on a crowded expressway generates a lot of tension. On top of that, as a driver you must sit in a position that strains your arms and shoulders, encourages you to thrust your head alertly forward, and forces you to remain in a fixed position for long periods. I consider myself lucky because my car has arm-rests on both sides of the driver's seat, allowing me to transfer some of the weight of my upper body to my elbows. That does a lot to reduce the stress on my shoulder muscles. An adjustable steering wheel also helps, if you can afford the car that goes with it. As for the fixed seating posture, there is no magic solution, but there are several things you can do. Avoid sitting so far back from the wheel that you must hold your arms straight out in front of you. Shift your body weight back and forth, sitting well forward now and then as a variation from your normal position. And, if you can, stop the car every hour or so to get out for a stretch and a short walk.

• A great deal of neck strain comes from reading in bed or from assuming a poor sleeping position. If you must read in bed, use some comfortable pillows to prop yourself up into a seated position. Make sure you can hold the book and see it comfortably without straining your neck, your shoulders, or your arms. Or buy a reading-stand that swings over the edge of the bed. Otherwise, do your reading in a comfortable chair before going to bed. That may not be the most convenient arrangement, but it's a small sacrifice to make for a pain-free neck.

As for sleeping in a poor position, many people have trouble if they sleep on their stomachs. For one thing, that position creates a sway back. Even worse, it forces you to twist your neck to one side, causing strain that may last all night. Another bad habit is sleeping with your head on a pillow so thick that it thrusts your head and neck forward when you lie on your back. The pillow should allow you to keep your head back between your shoulders, not jammed forward. I have found many people with neck pain have trouble with solid foam rubber pillows. I generally recommend using a pillow that will give with the weight of your head and not fight back. If you keep waking up in the morning with a painful or stiff neck, you might consider changing your pillow or even getting a special neck pillow of the type we discussed in Chapter 1. As I mentioned, it is used under the neck, not under the head, and is most effective when you lie on your back. The typical cervical pillow is firm, not spongy, and about four inches thick. Newer models, designed to allow side sleeping, require some trial and error. There are other alternatives as well: a few patients get good protection and pain relief by sleeping in soft collars or cloth ruffs.

What about using a collar to protect your neck when you are not sleeping?

Like a brace for the low back, a cervical collar acts to restrict movement and take over the normal function of the supporting muscles. Using a collar to carry the weight of your head when your neck is sore may seem like a good idea, but it leads to some difficult problems. Your neck muscles rapidly lose their strength and tone, so you become dependent on the collar. Putting a collar on is easy; getting rid of it again may require weeks of exercise and increased pain.

The neck collar is also a common source of psychological dependency. Patients with chronic neck pain frequently feel compelled to wear a single ruff fitted so loosely that it provides no support or restriction of motion. It's almost like a feeble gesture of security to mark their profound suffering.

However, a cervical support does have some value. I routinely prescribe one after neck surgery or for use in specific situations where neck pain is likely, such as riding on public transit or driving heavy equipment. If you've been advised to use a collar, try to wear it only when recommended by your doctor and for as brief a period as possible. By combining that protection with regular neck exercise to maintain muscle tone you can avoid one of the major blocks to rapid rehabilitation.

Aren't there some relaxant pills you can take to ease the muscle spasms in your neck?

There are. But, as we've seen, relaxants have limitations. The term is not wrong but, as I have said, it's misleading. I think of them as "people relaxants," because you can't say to yourself, "This muscle in my neck is tense, so I'll just relax it by taking a pill." The pill doesn't know which of your muscles you are concerned about; it will relax them all. For that reason, you shouldn't take this type of medication if you have to remain alert. Using one of those pills can be like taking a stiff drink: alcohol is the most widely used "people relaxant" of all.

However, if you are in a position to relax safely, and you need relief from pain brought on by muscular tension, the medication might be a good idea.

What about pain killers?

As I pointed out earlier, many of the so-called pain killers we use don't actually remove or block the pain but simply alter your perception of it. You still feel the pain but you don't care. The headache no longer bothers you so much – but then neither does anything else. When you combine a pain killer with a tranquilizer you certainly feel better, but you cannot expect to function normally. And that way of feeling better can be a problem in itself. It's easy to understand why some people get into the habit of handling their pain with medication instead of exercise and proper posture.

Used properly, relaxants and pain killers are just temporary remedies.

Do you recommend heat or ice packs to relieve neck pain?

As with back pain, both heat and cold can be useful. They are just two of many counter-irritants that "jam" the nervous system in much the same way as a shortwave broadcaster will jam an enemy's radio messages. When you use heat or cold or other irritants, the brain gets a strong impulse that blocks the pain signal. And so you feel heat or cold but not pain.

Sometimes even a violent counter-irritant can provide welcome relief. I have had neck pain off and on for years. One winter recently, for no apparent reason, I suffered an excruciating attack. For months it interfered with my work. The pain was predominantly along the inner border of my right shoulder blade. I could feel a muscle knot there that was extremely painful. At first I got good temporary relief from a strong back rub. Then I discovered that punching the muscle was even better, and so I would invite my teenaged son to hit my upper back as hard as he could – really pound it. The counter-irritant effect gave me some great pain-free moments. Unless you've been through it yourself, you might find it hard to believe what some of us will put up with to get even temporary relief.

Would it be fair to say that pounding on a painful knot of muscle is a form of manipulation?

No, although pounding and manipulation may both provide relief. When my son punched my knotted muscle, he was providing a counter-irritant, but he was not manipulating the spine. Manipulation refers to maneuvers that put the joints through a range of movement. For reasons no one fully understands, that sometimes relieves the spasm.

It may surprise you that when I took my problem to a physical therapist for manipulation, she ignored the back spasm and worked directly on my neck. If I'd had no medical knowledge, I would have expected her to start on that knotted muscle. But she was providing the correct treatment, gentle manual traction and manipulation. She performed this treatment by pulling up on my head with both hands while gently turning my neck to the left, away from the painful side. The action produced a faint cracking sound, but it didn't hurt.

Did the manipulation produce the results you were looking for?

After the first treatment, it was amazing. I had virtually no pain and I could move my neck any way I wanted. I hadn't realized how much I had been limiting my neck movement to avoid the pain.

Are you saying that after one session of physical therapy your neck pain was gone?

Temporarily, yes. But being a typical patient and a typical doctor, I got busy and ignored her instructions to come back within a day or two for more treatment. My pain returned, as bad as ever. After several days without treatment, I went back and had virtually the same treatment again. But this time it didn't help much. I got slight relief that lasted only a few hours. I never made it back for a third session. I simply waited it out, exercising very gently to strengthen the muscles and making the pain more bearable by assuming postures that reduced my discomfort.

So what do you think about manipulation as a remedy for neck pain?

When muscle tension is a major factor, manipulation can be very effective. As with my first treatment it can produce dramatic results. But it doesn't always work that well. Although it has been shown that manipulation can hasten recovery, it has never been proven to alter the final outcome. Manipulation provides no benefit if you are having no problems at the time it is performed. In other words, it relieves symptoms but does little or nothing to remedy the cause. That's why I tell patients there's no point in continuing to go back indefinitely for more treatments if your neck is no longer stiff or painful.

Is manipulation painful?

No, it isn't; or rather, it shouldn't be, if it is being used to relieve neck or back pain. In other areas it can hurt a great deal. We talked earlier about the way your shoulder may stiffen up with neck trouble or with an immobilized arm. This frozen shoulder can require some pretty drastic manipulation. In spite of what you may think, doctors don't usually employ a treatment that must hurt the patient in order to help him, but that's what must be done to restore mobility in a frozen shoulder.

Remember I described how the shoulder stiffens as parts of the capsule stick together? Occasionally the patient's shoulder becomes so bound up by that process that you have to put him under anesthetic and move the joint for him, literally tearing the adhesions while putting the arm through the movements the patient can't make on his own. The main shoulder movement to be restored is the motion someone makes when throwing a baseball. The manipulation is done with the patient lying on his back with his shoulder over the edge of the table. Usually you can hear the scar tissue tearing; it sounds like the crunching of footsteps in crusty snow. The patient feels nothing at the time, of course, although he wakes up with one very sore shoulder. But once the capsular folds have been separated and the range of shoulder movement restored, the patient has a chance to maintain the normal function and get rid of his pain.

Wouldn't such drastic manipulation of the shoulder aggravate the person's neck pain?

Not as a rule. Often, the neck pain which may have caused the shoulder problem in the first place has long since disappeared, and only the stiff shoulder remains to be treated. Besides, the neck is carefully protected, and this manipulation is limited to the normal range of shoulder movement.

Manipulation of the neck itself is not nearly as dramatic, but the objective is the same: to loosen stiff joints and regain normal movement. Just like the patient who has had a shoulder manipulated, you must exercise often after neck manipulation to keep your increased mobility until the discomfort disappears.

You said part of the physical therapy for your neck pain was "manual traction." What is manual traction and what does it do?

Traction for the neck means pulling on the head to stretch the muscles and ligaments around the cervical spine. In my case the traction was manual; that is, the therapist pulled only with her hands. Often, neck traction is applied mechanically, using a series of hanging weights. At professional clinics you'll find therapists using traction tables designed to apply adjustable or intermittent patterns of pull, either to the neck or to the low back. Like manipulation, traction is intended to reduce muscle spasm, to free up stiff joints, and, of course, relieve pain. Because the head only weighs about twenty pounds (9 kg), traction can slightly open the exit canals of the nerve roots between the vertebrae and put tension on the bulging outer shell of each disc. The situation is quite different here than in the much larger lumbar spine, where conventional traction produces little if any separation between the vertebrae.

For this reason, traction can be helpful in relieving Type Three (pinched nerve) pain in the neck. It also has some benefit in reducing Type Two pain from a bulging disc. In my case, the effect was mainly to relieve severe muscle spasm. Of course, the stretching action is temporary. Once the pull is released, the structures return to their normal positions.

Many people learn to use traction on their own at home. If you try it, remember that the position of your neck is important. A slight change in the amount of flexion or extension can make all the difference to the success of the treatment. If you decide to get your own traction equipment, be sure to obtain proper instruction as well.

As a victim of neck trouble yourself, what positions or movements have you found useful for pain relief?

I devised my own form of manual traction, pulling up on my head with both hands and gently turning it away from the side of pain. I found I could relieve the pain for several minutes that way, although I suspect I looked a little strange. Because I have Type Two pain, a second useful maneuver consisted of arching my neck backward. I would lie on my back with my head hanging over the edge of a bed and a small pillow under the nape of my neck. This position minimized the pressure on the discs in my cervical spine and reduced my pain.

If my symptoms had come from worn facet joints, I would likely have found comfort by hanging my head forward to relieve the load on those small joints in the back of my spine. Because there is more than one cause of neck pain there is no single position that will help everyone. It is possible to distinguish Type One from Type Two pain in the neck just as we can in the low back, but finding the right movement or posture for your own pain is a matter of careful experimentation.

What can I do to improve my posture to relieve my neck pain?

Here's a technique I recommend to most of my patients. Start by imagining that your head is being picked up like a melon on a fruit vendor's stand; now, without actually touching it with your hands, lift it up, move it back, and place it squarely between your shoulders. The maneuver takes a little practice but it's worth learning. It's a good way of counteracting the habit most of us develop of standing and sitting with the head thrust forward, a posture that produces considerable strain on the neck. If you consciously try to position your head directly over your shoulders, your muscle tension will decrease noticeably. Some people, misunderstanding the technique, tilt their heads back and look up – which is wrong. Your head should move back without tilting, and your line of vision should remain level.

That principle is especially important if you are engaged in some activity that keeps you seated for a long period. Whether you are working at a desk, watching television, reading a book, or driving your car, do whatever is necessary to avoid thrusting your neck forward. That may mean finding a different chair or a better way to sit. It may mean discarding your bifocal glasses in some situations where you would otherwise tilt your head back so as to see through the lower lenses. Many people with personal computers have this problem, and the smart ones are getting single-lens reading glasses especially for use at their video display terminals.

Whatever it takes, make proper posture one of your regular habits and you'll be doing a lot to relieve or ward off neck pain.

I gather it takes a lot of conscious effort at first.

That's right. Start by thinking, right now, about how you are holding your body, especially about the position of your neck. Keep concentrating on correcting your posture until the right habits become second nature.

Meanwhile, remember that your neck, like the rest of your body, has its limitations, and if you push it beyond those limits, you're asking for trouble.

Once you establish that awareness, you'll be surprised how often you find simple ways of changing a familiar routine to eliminate discomfort or pain. I learned that lesson when I started scuba diving. Each time I came out of the water, I had a nasty headache. At first I assumed the problem occurred because of the difference between the pressure under water and the normal atmospheric pressure at the surface. But then I noticed that if I only looked at the bottom while I was diving, my headache wouldn't be so bad. I suddenly realized my scuba apparatus was to blame. I had been wearing a type of buoyancy compensator that fits around the neck like a yoke on an ox. It pulled my neck down and forced me to strain upward whenever I wanted to see where I was going. With the next dive, I switched to a stabilization jacket – an inflatable vest that serves the same purpose but places no strain on the neck. As soon as I made that switch, my scuba-diving headaches disappeared.

What about exercise as a means of preventing neck pain? Is that a good idea?

Exercise is not just a good idea; it's a *must*. But there is an irony worth noting here, for all those who exercise to protect themselves from low-back pain. One primary objective in back exercise is to strengthen the abdominal muscles, and this is often done by practicing sit-ups.

The trouble is that when people with weak stomach muscles try to do a sit-up, they invariably raise their heads off the mat first. They use the muscles of their necks and upper back, often pulling forward with their hands behind their heads as well, to help generate the force they need to raise their upper bodies. Now if they happen to have neck problems, particularly from worn and bulging discs, the added stress from this action will produce a very sore neck.

People with low-back problems must learn to do their sit-ups properly – literally to save their necks. The correct way is to keep your head back on top of your shoulders and raise your whole upper body as a unit. That keeps the strain off the neck and places it where it belongs – on the abdominal muscles.

I want to emphasize that exercise of any kind is *not* right for someone with acute neck pain. You should treat an acute attack here as you would treat acute pain anywhere else in your spine: gently. Later, when the pain subsides, return to your exercises.

If you do them regularly, you'll quite likely find future attacks are less severe and will subside a lot faster.

It's important to remember that exercise goes hand in hand with the other measures I suggested earlier – the various habits and tricks you can adopt to achieve proper posture and avoid tension and stress. In a nutshell, these are all ways of achieving and maintaining a neck that's strong enough to handle the tasks it's called upon to perform.

My advice will disappoint anyone who is looking for magic answers or spectacular forms of treatment, but it happens to be the best advice I can provide, and it has one great thing going for it: it usually works.

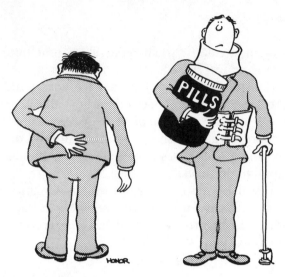

6. BACK PATIENT OR PAIN PATIENT?

Are you a *back* patient or a *pain* patient? There is a very important distinction.

If your primary problem is pain originating from a physical condition in your spine, you are a back patient. But if that *same* back pain has taken over your life, dictating your daily activities and influencing your every decision, you are no longer just a back patient but a pain patient as well.

To illustrate how you can get that way, I'll tell you about three back patients who became pain patients.

One is a woman I'll call Freda Kovacs, now forty-three. Late one afternoon about five years ago, she was offered a ride home from the factory where she worked as a sewing-machine operator. As the car waited for a red light to change, it was struck from behind by another vehicle.

Mrs. Kovacs went to hospital for X-rays and was told there was nothing wrong. The X-rays of her spine showed only the amount of wear and tear normal for her age. But within a day or two, her neck began to ache. She saw her own doctor, who eventually prescribed a full array of pills – pain killers, muscle relaxants, anti-inflammatory drugs, and tranquilizers. In spite of her repeated visits to complain of the pain, they were the only treatment she ever received.

After several weeks at home she went back to work. But even with the medication, she couldn't operate her sewing machine without suffering. She quit her job and began to withdraw from the world. First, she stopped seeing friends, then she quit doing housework. Her husband and two teenaged daughters took over her chores. Freda Kovacs had become a full-time invalid.

I met her only recently, when I was asked to examine her in connection with the lawsuit arising from the accident. In all the standard tests for diagnosing back pain, no physical cause could be discovered. Her muscle strength is normal. So are her reflexes. She has no nerve irritation. The list goes on. Everything checks out normally. There is nothing physically wrong with Freda Kovacs. And yet, no question about it, this woman is suffering genuine pain.

Why? I'm convinced it's mainly because she sees herself as a disabled person. And she got that way because she was a victim of inadequate care. Her case was regarded as a purely physical problem, and was treated with techniques that were entirely passive; no one attempted to involve Mrs. Kovacs in any part of her own recovery. She needed help with the emotional distress she suffered after the car accident. It's quite likely that with the right encouragement and reassurance, along with the proper physical training, she would have returned to her job much sooner than she did, and stuck it out until the pain subsided.

Now, I'm afraid, it's too late. Freda Kovacs, the victim of an accident that was physically inconsequential, has become permanently disabled.

In the second case, my patient was a woman who, along with her husband, had been a social acquaintance of mine for several years. She was suffering from a pinched nerve in her low back. After seven months of unsuccessful treatment, she came to me for the first time, hopeful that my professional skill and our friendship would somehow combine to produce rapid relief from her pain. After considering various alternatives, we agreed to try an injection of chymopapain, which often eliminates the pressure from a bulging disc that causes Type Three pain. But in her case the injection didn't work, and at that point she exploded with all the frustration and rage that had built up inside her through eight months of pain.

I can't remember an occasion when anyone took more trouble to enunciate a complete, unabridged list of my shortcomings as a doctor: I didn't care about her. I had callously excluded her from the process of making decisions about her treatment. I had not even asked her opinion. I was supposed to be making her well but I had done nothing to help her.... She went on and on.

I just sat there, biting my tongue and reminding myself of the things I teach my medical students about responding to pain patients. The physician is not there to win an argument; he is there to help. There are no marks for outwitting or out-shouting the patient. But how much more comfortable it is to advocate that approach in class than to follow it in practice!

And I really don't blame that woman for behaving as she did. If you'd been through months of agony and frustration with still no relief in sight, wouldn't you take it out on any doctor who failed to help you get well?

I know the feeling. I've been through emotionally destructive pain myself – not from my chronic back condition but from a form of recurrent migraine known as a cluster headache, which plagued me for years. The pain would fill my eyes with tears until I couldn't see and it would pound inside my skull until I couldn't stand still. Under those conditions, how can you possibly remain your normal, amiable self? Your whole personality changes, while you live in fear between bouts, waiting for the pain to erupt once more.

Obviously, that experience has given me a perspective on pain I never learned in medical school. I can look at someone in pain and say, "Yes, I understand what you're telling me." And understanding certainly helped me endure the tirade directed at me by that patient whose problem I had not yet solved.

Fortunately, that stormy session ended on a cheerful note. Having vented her rage, she felt better, and we knew where we stood with each other. Since then, we have moved ahead with effective treatment.

In the third case, I declined to accept the individual as my patient. My only contact with the man was a letter he wrote from another city to ask whether I would diagnose the back pain that had troubled him constantly for twelve and a half years. That time period alone told me he was far beyond the stage of simple physical back pain. It was reason enough to refer him for pain management. But there was more – significantly more. With his letter he had enclosed a loose-leaf binder containing a neatly typewritten, fifty-five-page monograph entitled "A Patient's Perspective of His Own Back Pain." It came complete with appendixes and a short bibliography. The poor man had become so obsessed with his back pain that he was making a career of analyzing it.

In response, I put him in touch with a pain clinic not far from his city, pointing out that the assessment he had asked for was the easy part; the big problem lay in controlling his chronic pain.

Although they reacted differently, all three of these patients have significant pain problems. My patient with the failed chymopapain injection had developed a strong emotional reaction that was beginning to change her personality and intensify her pain. The others had already crossed the line separating two types of pain victims: those with persistent physical pain, which is bad enough, and those who have had the greater misfortune of being entrapped by CPS – chronic pain syndrome.

In this chapter I describe the syndrome and offer practical advice which I hope will help some back patients avoid becoming pain patients.

I went to my doctor to see what could be done about my back pain but he couldn't find anything wrong with me. Now I'm wondering whether my family is right when they say I'm just imagining the pain. What do you think?

I can tell you one thing without even examining you: if you feel pain, it's real. The idea that you are imagining the whole thing is based on a common misconception about pain. Many people assume that if pain has no physical cause, you can't really be feeling anything, and your distress is somehow imaginary. But that's not true. Pain can be caused by many, many factors – physical and emotional. And they interact. The cycle usually, though not necessarily, starts with a physical cause, such as an injury. We react emotionally to the pain, and that emotion itself contributes more pain. Our reaction causes the muscles to tense, thereby introducing another physical factor – the spasm. And then we react emotionally to the spasm, and so it goes, around and around in a vicious, self-perpetuating loop.

Even after the initiating physical cause has disappeared, the pain may continue, triggered by those emotional responses.

Is that psychogenic pain?

Yes. Psychogenic pain is the technical term for pain produced by an emotional response without an accompanying physical cause; literally, pain generated by the psyche. Unfortunately the phrase is often used when the examiner doesn't believe the patient actually feels pain. And that's not correct. As I've just explained, pain originating in the mind is as real as the pain from bodily injury. Pain is pain no matter where it starts.

I wish everyone would realize that when the doctor says, "I can't find anything wrong with you" he's not necessarily accusing you of lying about your pain. What he is saying is that the cause of your trouble doesn't appear to be physical. Obviously he would allay your concerns more readily if he clarified the basis for diagnosing physical pain in one case and psychogenic pain in another. Often it's a matter of determining whether the initial cause was structural or not and whether that original cause still exists. He should help you recognize that a combination of factors may be involved – fear, anxiety, anger, depression, and various other emotions – plus muscular tension, stress, and fatigue.

Your doctor can provide a good service by exploring those additional features of the problem with you, particularly if he finds that your pain has no apparent physical origin. He will try to learn whether you have been upset about anything lately, or have been under any unusual pressure. One inevitable pressure that is often overlooked is the burden of the pain itself. Other events may intensify the problem, the way a door-slam will when you have a headache, but the very presence of the headache is enough to make you upset.

Questions in this area need to be asked in such a way that you will understand how natural and commonplace it is to feel pain that has no significant physical cause. Otherwise, the doctor's mention of emotional problems might trigger another false assumption on your part – that psychogenic pain is a symptom of mental disorders: "My god! The doctor thinks I'm losing my mind!" And, of course, that's not what's meant either.

Are you saying that people's aches and pains are *never* imaginary?

Of course there are hypochondriacs and hysterics, who react to imaginary pain. But they are rare – more rare than many people suppose – and they, too, are suffering from real diseases, forms of mental illness that can be just as disabling as the chronic pain syndrome.

But you said a person may keep on feeling pain from an injury after it heals. Isn't that the same as imaginary pain?

No, that's not the same thing. During the time the injury is there, your body develops a "memory" that may keep the pain alive after the injury has healed. If your muscles have learned how to spasm and hurt, anything that tightens those muscles in the same way – it might be fatigue, emotional tension, or even a cold draft – can trigger that pain all over again.

It's possible, too, for a person to be conditioned to feel pain merely because he or she *expects* to feel it. I actually test for this reaction whenever I examine someone with long-standing back pain. One method I use is to rotate the patient's trunk by moving his hip joints. The patient stands with both feet on the floor while I hold his arms to his sides and twist his pelvis. This movement places no stress whatever on the spine, and yet often a chronic pain sufferer will cry out with back pain. This reaction is a sign that the person expects to feel back pain (or thinks I am expecting him to feel it) and so he actually experiences the pain on cue.

One of my patients complains of numbness all down one side of his body, although he has nothing physically wrong with him. Even though there can be no purely organic cause to produce such a problem, I accept it as a genuine complaint. I do believe, however, that he exaggerates the condition, either consciously or otherwise, because he's afraid that without it I might fail to recognize the "seriousness" of his condition.

I sympathize with a patient who behaves that way. I know what chronic pain does to you, and I think it's all too easy for someone who has never had the problem to unjustly accuse the victim of exaggeration. There is simply no way to tell what some other person is actually feeling.

But that does bring up the question of malingering, which means lying about having an illness. It can be difficult to determine whether a patient is actually experiencing the pain he describes or just trying to fool the examiner for some gain, such as an increased disability settlement. Although many people exaggerate their problem, very few make the whole thing up. The factor that often decides the issue is consistency both in response to the examination and in everyday life. The patient who winces and screams with every movement in the office, and then dashes out to put another quarter in the parking meter, deserves to be viewed with suspicion.

Occasionally, a colleague of mine who runs a pain clinic in Vancouver asks a group of patients to line up along one wall of the room and then arrange themselves according to who feels the most pain – the worst in one corner and then the rest in descending order. Invariably, this request creates a small stampede. Everybody in the class tries to get into the corner reserved for those with the worst pain.

Their reaction to that test is typical of chronic pain patients everywhere, and it's not hard to see why. After all, each person has what he can truthfully describe as "100 percent of my own pain." And whatever that 100 percent amounts to, it's as much pain as its owner ever wants to have – and often as much as he thinks he can stand.

Obviously, pain is a very individual and subjective thing.

That's right. It's also very complicated. Perhaps you were taught in health class that you feel pain simply because a nerve in some part of your body sends a pain signal to your brain. That's the traditional concept. But in recent years, medical researchers have found that the process is not that simple. The signal that is sent is not necessarily the message the brain receives. The message is changed as it travels – changed in the spinal cord and changed again in the brain itself. Although we don't understand how some of these changes happen, we know there are many things that can affect the intensity of pain.

I would think that my attitude has a bearing on the way pain affects me.

You're right, it does. The amount you suffer from a bout of pain depends on a great many factors: the mood you are in, the amount of sleep you had last night, whether you and your mate are getting along well, how the "vibes" are in the office, and so on. You can be sure your chronic backache will feel a lot worse on the day your lose your wallet than it will on the day you win ten thousand dollars in a lottery.

Your perception of pain also depends partly on the efficiency of your sensory system. You have heard of people who can somehow stand a lot more pain than the rest of us – professional athletes, for instance. The quarterback who goes back into the game in spite of a broken finger is using inner resources we can't measure or even define. He may be particularly good at blocking out pain signals by concentrating on his game. Or he may simply be one of those people with a high tolerance to pain. In that case he is not any braver than the rest of us – he just suffers less because his pain transport system is less efficient or less sensitive than normal.

Is pain tolerance something that improves with practice?

No, just the opposite. Each of us has a finite ability to endure pain. The longer we are forced to cope with the problem the less reserve we have left, like a car running out of gas.

Once our tolerance is exhausted, even a minor pain produces great suffering. That's why a pain that actually remains unchanged over several months will become harder and harder to bear, and may be perceived as growing worse.

I gather you don't use the terms "pain" and "suffering" to mean the same thing.

No, doctors make a useful distinction between the two.

Pain is what results when that signal is transmitted from the hurt part of your body through your spinal cord to your brain.

Suffering describes what you, as an individual, do with that pain – how you perceive it and what effect it has on your emotional state. You may have a lot of pain and suffer very little, or you may have a small amount of pain and suffer a great deal.

People who suffer a lot from a small amount of discomfort or pain naturally become known as complainers. I've noticed that, often, when two people catch the same flu bug at the same time, one person will suffer more – or certainly complain more. But who can say the complainer is not actually feeling much worse than the other person? It's a very subjective thing, and we have no way of measuring it.

And while we're on terminology, there's a third word to mention: disability. Whereas suffering has to do with our perception of pain, disability refers to the way our behavior is altered in response to that suffering. Disability has an element of objectivity we don't find in the other two terms. It is objective because we can all see the changes in someone's pattern of activity. We may not be able to measure pain or suffering, but we can certainly count the number of days a patient stays off work.

Disability has a subjective aspect as well, since two individuals with the same problem may handle it quite differently. When two people have similar leg injuries, one person may walk with a slight limp, minimizing the difficulty as much as possible, while the other may hobble around on crutches.

That second person is in danger of acquiring a learned dis- ability – an unfortunate phenomenon that is all too common. I once had a patient who told me with some pride that he had learned to live with his bad back and that he needed no further treatment. He no longer worked and no longer took part in any active recreation. He spent at least six hours a day in bed resting, and when he wasn't in bed he was still indoors, "caring" for his back.

Contrary to what he said, this man had not learned to control his back problem. He had learned how to be disabled. His problem was no longer his pain or his suffering. His problem was "learned helplessness," a pattern of behaving like an invalid, which he had taught himself through years of practice.

You have spoken repeatedly about chronic pain but you haven't mentioned acute pain. Does acute pain present the same kinds of problems?

Not really. Acute pain occurs quite predictably from illness or injury. If you break a leg, it's bound to be painful. The pain may last for weeks or even months, but acute pain is recognized by the patient as having a definite end point. It will disappear as the injury mends. Since we know we can eliminate acute pain by treating its cause, we don't usually treat the pain behavior, although we may provide medication to relieve the suffering.

Chronic pain, on the other hand, is pain that persists for six months or longer; a nagging backache, for instance. The patient begins to worry that the pain will never end but will persist for the rest of his life. Whether or not it ever had a physical origin, chronic pain often becomes an entity – and a problem – separate from the cause. For that reason, doctors, as well as treating the source, will often treat chronic pain independently.

One special difficulty with chronic pain arises when an acute organic cause, such as a sore joint in the spine, subsides but remains sufficiently irritable to trigger local muscle spasms and pain; or when the "memory" factor I mentioned comes into play. In either case, the actual physical problem is so minor there is nothing we can do about it. So we try to treat the pain itself. That's not impossible, but it's difficult because there are a lot of things we have yet to learn about managing pain. If we knew more, we might encounter fewer cases of people whose pain problem has progressed so far that it has become incurable.

Is there some specific point at which you can say, "This patient's pain is incurable"?

Yes, but I'm afraid with our present state of knowledge and lack of sophistication in treating chronic pain, we can't precisely identify when the transition takes place. In time, however, some patients will reach a point where, in my opinion, they are beyond help,

even from the most highly skilled pain specialists. Our understanding of pain management today is comparable to our knowledge of tuberculosis half a century ago, when we treated that
affliction simply with fresh air, sunshine, and rest. A great deal
depends on the natural course of the disease.

A woman I'll call Hilda Carson is someone I remember well
as a pain patient who was beyond help. A woman in her early
fifties, she had been working as a mature model and a part-time
clerk. Her problem began in the store where she worked. One
day, she climbed a ladder to retrieve some stock from a high
shelf, fell, and broke her left heel.

By the time I saw her she had already been through three
rounds of surgery – one attempt to correct the original injury, and
two others to fuse some of the damaged joints in the foot.

She hobbled into my office with a cane and told me her whole
story. By now, the pain, originally confined to her heel, was surging
through the entire foot and beginning to radiate into her lower
leg, knee, and buttock. My examination showed that the operations
had accomplished all that could be done to help her and more
surgery would be of no value. Mrs. Carson was left with a chronically
painful heel.

But I could see also that her pain was no longer entirely physical,
since her symptoms far exceeded what you could expect from
the original injury. I encouraged her to tell me more about herself
and her problems. At the time of the accident, she had been
happily married. But because of her heel pain, she didn't want
to make love. She and her husband were soon quarreling, and
eventually he left her. According to Hilda, he treated her badly
in the financial settlement.

Now here she was, into her fifties, beginning to look sixty, trying
hard to look forty, and unable to work as a model or a clerk.
And, given her emotional state and physical problems, she was
unlikely to be hired or accepted for training in any job.

As she said, "Who's going to hire a middle-aged cripple with
a cane?"

And she was probably right. She had come to see herself as
a totally disabled person, and for good reason. By now, her physical
condition was almost incidental to the economic, social, and
emotional problems it had spawned. Her broken marriage, her
poverty, her inability to find work, her loneliness, her sense of

despair – all these had combined to make her a classic victim of the chronic pain syndrome.

We discussed the nature of her pain, and I tried to help her understand what was happening. But she wasn't interested. If I couldn't take away her suffering with my surgery, she would find someone else. I don't often see a patient whose problems leave me feeling absolutely helpless, but that's how I felt after seeing Hilda Carson.

Is it usually fairly obvious when a person's pain problem is emotional rather than physical?

Often, but not always. Emotion, like pain itself, is not something you can measure. Sometimes it's hard to identify a patient's real emotions and then determine how much those emotions are contributing to the problem. Not long ago I saw a woman in her sixties who appeared to be coping very well with a chronic back disorder, even though it had severely limited her life. She had given up most of the things she enjoyed: bowling, gardening, ballroom dancing. She now spent much of her time looking after her invalid husband, who was confined to their home after a stroke.

Although those nursing duties aggravated her back pain, she didn't complain. In fact, she described her whole situation in a fairly calm, matter-of-fact way.

Then I began questioning her more specifically about the way her circumstances were curtailing her normal activities. At that point she broke down and cried. Abruptly, her whole manner changed. Even her choice of words was different. She was no longer speaking by rote, in the calm language she had taught herself to use when discussing her situation with friends. The extent to which she had shut the problem out of her mind became clear when she suddenly blurted out, "I only cry when I think about it."

I couldn't help feeling that a lot of her back pain came from the suppression of her emotions: the unhappiness, the anger, and the resentment she felt over the things that were happening to her. Again, here was a heavy overlay of emotion complicating a problem that was initially physical. But few, if any, of those secondary factors would be evident to anyone who engaged that woman in only casual conversation.

Is there a difference between any long-lasting pain and the chronic pain syndrome?

It is sometimes difficult to distinguish one from the other during a first consultation, but there is a crucial difference. The chronic pain syndrome – call it CPS – is a behavioral disorder. It is characterized by certain components and conditions that don't generally apply to patients who are coping with a lengthy but resolving pain problem and are able to continue functioning normally. These CPS characteristics include: pain of suspiciously long duration; pain that's out of proportion to the physical findings; the diagnosis of a soft-tissue injury; a gradually expanding array of symptoms; a preoccupation with physical complaints; "pill-popping"; "doctor-shopping"; a failure to respond to conventional treatment; a loss of sex drive; and various changes in the patient's personality and emotional makeup. These last factors usually cause marital and family problems, as they did for Hilda Carson with her broken heel.

Would you elaborate on the signs and symptoms of CPS?

All right. The first point I mentioned is, pain of suspiciously long duration. By that I mean a period of at least six months. You may have a pain that has lasted longer than you expected, but if it has been bothering you for only a week, or even a month, there's no reason to be frightened or to worry about the syndrome. Even after six months, you may have a pain that occurs only when you do a certain thing, such as putting your full weight on an ankle that was sprained and is still mending. In this kind of situation, the pain is not a result of CPS, but just the reflection of local irritation from a condition that is taking a long time to heal. With the syndrome you have pain in excess of anything indicated by the physical findings. You may even have begun to wonder whether the pain really is "all your head," as your family and friends have been saying. Most patients with CPS, however, cling stubbornly to the idea that their problem has a real and, usually, serious physical cause. In either case, the doctor can find no objective evidence of a specific impairment, such as true weakness, or loss of a reflex. The doctor detects little or nothing out of order, certainly nothing to justify the pain you are experiencing.

Again I emphasize that it's not a question of whether the pain is real; we know that if you are feeling pain, it *is* real. But by now the pain itself is not even the problem. The real problem is your *response* to that pain. With CPS, the degree and the nature of that response are excessive – that is, inappropriate – for your trouble.

Don't confuse this exaggerated response with malingering. The latter is a conscious decision, a lie, aimed at fooling someone. The chronic pain response produces real pain and real disability even though there isn't much physically wrong for the doctor to see.

Apparently there is some important point to be made as well about a soft-tissue injury as opposed to, say, a broken bone.

Yes. As I pointed out earlier, a fracture may take a long time to heal and continue causing pain for the duration. But if you suffer a soft-tissue injury, such as a pulled muscle or a bruise, you shouldn't be feeling constant pain from it after six months or so. Soft-tissue injuries heal much faster than that. Of course, there will be no sign of injury in your X-rays and, as I mentioned, no other positive indications from objective observations or tests. A patient's undue concern with simple soft-tissue injury can be the first step towards a serious chronic pain problem.

This is particularly true when we consider back pain because the element of fear is so great. A sprained spinal joint or a herniated disc will heal just as other soft-tissue injuries do, but the unnecessary worry over a "bad back" can linger on and lead to trouble.

You said the chronic pain syndrome is a disorder. Does that mean it's a disease in itself?

Yes. It *is* a disease – a behavioral disease – and it needs to be treated as such. It must also be clearly separated from mental illness. The excessive response and the development of an invalid behavior pattern can happen solely as a result of persistent pain without any other psychiatric problems. The abnormally increased awareness of pain in CPS is clearly emphasized by the next item on my list: an increasing number of symptoms. In other words, the pain tends to spread. The problem may develop in your back, but the next thing you know your whole body seems to hurt. You get frequent headaches, tingling sensations in your arms and legs, sore joints, chest pains, and many tender lumps in the muscles over the shoulders and at the back of the pelvis. To make matters worse, you now focus even more of your attention on these bodily aches and pains. The situation is especially difficult if you also happen to have a minor physical difficulty such as mild disc pain. Your whole lifestyle begins to center on these problems and you may talk or think about little else. Everything you do is weighed against the effect it will have on your pain. "I'd love to go boating tonight, but I'm afraid it might hurt my back...."

Along with this expanding array of symptoms you may experience general fatigue and probably insomnia. In fact, sleep disruption is almost an inevitable feature of the chronic pain syndrome.

You don't mean to say that if back pain keeps me awake at night I must have CPS.

Certainly not. Pain that disturbs your sleep is most likely to be just ordinary backache, and if it bothers you night after night, you may develop a pattern of sleeping poorly. Pain of this sort characteristically gets worse any time you overuse your back, and that can make getting to sleep even more difficult.

On the other hand, if there is no apparent relationship between your pain and your activity, and if pain is a major problem whenever you try to rest, your doctor will want to see whether you might have one of the rare physical causes of constant back pain, such as a bone tumor. Of course that's most unlikely.

My point is simply that insomnia, which troubles some back patients for obvious reasons, is usually a part of the chronic pain syndrome as well.

**You said that victims of the syndrome are often "pill-poppers."
Isn't it likely that these people tended to overuse medication even before they developed chronic pain?**

I don't think so. We're not talking about an illness that affects only people with weak personalities who go through life looking for psychological crutches to lean on. While it's true that some victims are people who would probably dote on a medical problem of any kind, they are not typical. The chronic pain syndrome is something that can happen to anybody – just as a ruptured disc or sore joint can. Never underestimate the power of pain. I know what it can do to people. As the "bad guys" like to say in the torture scenes you read in spy novels, everybody has a breaking point. A lot of people have reached that breaking point before they ever set foot in my office. It doesn't surprise me that they have become pill-poppers. And it depresses me to think of how many of them got that way because a doctor prescribed medication as their only form of treatment. In many instances the patients have become completely irrational about it.

What's irrational about taking pills to relieve pain?

Nothing, if they help. But often the first words I hear are, "You've got to help me, Doctor, because I'm taking all these pills, and nothing seems to work."

"Then why do you take the pills," I ask, "if they don't work?"

"Well, I've got all this pain."

"But you just said the pills don't help. And if they don't help, why do you take them?"

"Actually, I've tried stopping, but I have to take them because of all this pain."

But isn't the person trying to tell you that without the pills the pain would be even worse?

That's a reasonable assumption, but often that's not how the chronic pain patient sees it. I ask, "On a scale of one to ten, with ten as the worst, how would you rate your pain when you use your medicine?"

"It's a ten – the worst."

"And how bad is it if you stop taking the pills?"

"Well, it's even worse!"

I sympathize with anyone in that situation, but this response only demonstrates the patient's inability to see his own problem with any sense of perspective: pain that is already "the worst" gets even worse if the pills are stopped. It has all the absurdity of those TV commercials for a washday detergent that somehow made your laundry "whiter than white."

Another thing these people fail to realize is that by taking all that medication they are getting into a vicious circle: *Why do I take the pills? Because I feel pain. Why do I feel pain? Because I'm sick. What makes me so sure I'm sick? I must be sick – look at all the pills I'm taking!*

For some CPS patients, the cycle is now complete and the treatment has become the reason for the disease which requires the treatment.

What is "doctor-shopping" and why is it part of the syndrome?

At first glance it seems obvious that patients with the chronic pain syndrome come to the doctor to get help. In a sense that's true, but typically they demand help strictly on their own terms. They don't want to hear the facts unless those facts fit their perception of their own disability. When the first doctor fails, they try a second, and then a third, and so on. They go the rounds and soon they're caught up in the system. It's all part of being sick – and of course they genuinely perceive themselves as sick people. Sick people need doctors, and so they keep finding new doctors to see. They become expert at manipulating the situation, playing one doctor off against another while remaining trapped on their own terrible treadmill.

Recently, after spending a great deal of time explaining the nature of his problem to a patient who was suffering from the chronic pain syndrome, I referred him to an excellent pain clinic. I emphasized to him that this local clinic could provide exactly the treatment he needed. After one visit to the clinic the man came back to tell me the director had found my diagnosis was completely wrong. I telephoned the clinic director, who said the patient told them I had diagnosed a serious problem of scar tissue in the spine, which would make it impossible for the clinic to help him. Both the clinic and I had come to the same conclusion about the patient. But since our opinions didn't match his own assessment, he was trying to manipulate us into a different course of action.

Just the other day, a woman came into my office for her second visit in a month. On her first, I had advised her to stop seeing doctors, including myself, to avoid passive treatments that offered only temporary relief from pain, and to begin a regular exercise program. But she had ignored that advice and had gone to see two other doctors. One had prescribed massage. The other was an acupuncturist who stuck needles into her. Because both practitioners had, in effect, offered to take charge of her problems while allowing her to passively await the results, she liked their treatments much better than my advice. Yet here she was, back in my office, saying, "Well, your last bit of advice was no help. What are you going to do for me now?" I felt as though she had dealt me into a round of poker and was challenging me to up the ante.

Do doctors try to discourage this kind of shopping around?

Yes, we do. Obviously it's a waste of our time – and a waste of the community's medical resources.

But can't it be argued that a patient has the right to seek a second opinion?

Yes – every right. And a third opinion, too, for that matter. But when a patient goes to half a dozen doctors complaining of the same condition and then ignores each one's advice if it doesn't appeal to him – that's doctor-shopping, pure and simple. Each doctor may have a different idea of the most appropriate treatment. But that's hardly grounds for the patient to go the rounds again, telling each doctor what a failure he is compared to the others. Yet that's typical of a patient with CPS.

You said that chronic pain patients don't get better with conventional treatment.

That's right, and they often prolong their treatments to extremes. It's not unusual in these cases to see physical therapy visits for deep heat and massage extending over a year or more. And I remember one woman who was carrying so many pills that her purse rattled. In any case, it's a mistake to apply the conventional techniques of acute pain management to patients suffering from CPS. Conventional management of acute, self-limiting pain is aimed mainly at the physical problem, and that's not where the real trouble lies in CPS. More important, conventional treatment is largely passive; it doesn't require the patient to do anything or take any responsibility for getting well. Given that kind of treatment, the CPS patient is more inclined to devote all his or her energy to remaining sick.

You mentioned a loss of sex drive as one of the syndrome's components. Does that affect men more often than women?

No – the actual loss of libido seems to afflict both sexes equally. A man may feel more devastated by the experience, but if it threatens or wrecks a marriage, as it did in the case of my "middle-aged cripple with a cane," it is obviously a serious problem for victims of both sexes and their mates.

Loss of libido can be devastating whatever the cause, but associated with CPS it introduces a whole new loop: if you lose your sex drive, you become anxious. Your anxiety is reflected in increased awareness of your problem, which intensifies your pain, which then perpetuates your loss of libido. Understandably, many CPS victims see this development as a sex problem, rather than as a byproduct of their pain. Consequently, they get into sex counseling when their actual need is to learn chronic pain management. It's hard for them to realize that once they conquer their pain their anxiety will be reduced and their libido will return.

Apart from sexual problems, how big a factor is anxiety in the syndrome?

It's a big factor, and it's just one of many emotions that keep the victim off balance and unable to lead a normal life. Anxiety is almost inevitable, and so are fear, anger, resentment – plus almost any other negative emotions you can think of. And, worst of all, these emotions are not just momentary, as they usually are for the rest of us, but they become part of the person's mood, night and day, to the point where the whole personality changes.

Even if I had never encountered a CPS case professionally, I could testify personally to some of those effects – although, at the time, I didn't realize how significant they were. Early in my career, I took a year of training in Scotland. As it happened, I arrived there during a severe bout of cluster headaches, which, this time, lasted nine weeks. Every day began with four hours of excruciating pain. Although it was gone before noon, I knew it would be back the next day, and that really got to me. Months later, long after the attacks were finished, several of my new friends there told me, "You are quite a different person from what you were when you first arrived," and "We see a tremendous difference in you since we first met."

Apparently they attributed this "tremendous difference" to the bracing climate of the Highlands. In reality, I had arrived in the country fighting off that terrible migraine pain. Without realizing it, I had reacted to the pain by becoming withdrawn, humorless, uncommunicative, even rude and hostile. Then, once my headaches subsided, I returned to normal, obviously impressing my Scottish friends with my "new" personality. I demonstrated many of the characteristics I now see in the CPS victims who come to me as patients. Almost without exception they are self-centered, demanding, intolerant, and very unhappy. They are so obsessed with their pain that they have built entire new – and miserable – lives around it, allowing it to dominate every moment of their time while forcing their families and friends to cater to its tyranny.

I was fortunate; my pain didn't last long enough to take over my life to that extent. But if I hadn't gone through some of that experience I would have great difficulty realizing that most people who now come to me with CPS are normally cheerful, likable individuals – and will be again, if they manage to escape the syndrome. Treatment isn't easy but it is possible.

Suppose I suspect my problem is chronic pain syndrome – how can I go about getting the right kind of help?

Begin by finding a doctor you feel comfortable with – somebody to whom you can tell your story. If your doctor doesn't seem interested, you should look elsewhere.

If you see a specialist, make sure that it is someone who is willing to discuss aspects of your problem that lie outside his or her specialty. If you are choosing a surgeon, for example, you will be better off selecting one who will recognize and discuss your emotional problem as well, even if he or she is unable to treat it.

Don't be afraid to ask questions. Make sure you understand the nature and purpose of the tests and treatments prescribed for you. There should be no mystery about anything that's being done.

Look for thoroughness. You don't want a doctor or therapist or chiropractor giving you a hasty examination and deciding, on little or no evidence, that there's nothing wrong with you except your pain. If you do get a speedy diagnosis, you need to know that it's backed by plenty of knowledge and skill. Whatever the treatment – a special diet, manipulation, an injection, or something else – it must be tailored exactly to suit your diagnosis and your personal situation. Treatment-by-rote just isn't good enough.

Look for a doctor who encourages you to assume a positive outlook and suggests something for you to do to help yourself. You will greatly increase your chances of dealing successfully with chronic pain if you assume as much responsibility as you can and take control of the situation to the fullest extent possible.

It may seem logical to expect a doctor to provide you with medical care just the way you expect a mechanic to provide your car with service. It's perfectly reasonable to drive into a garage and say, "My brakes aren't working properly. Please see what's wrong and fix it." A mechanic who's skilled and conscientious will do as you ask, without any help from you.

But the medical treatment of chronic pain doesn't work that way. You can't expect to get well simply by handing your problem to a doctor and saying, "Here it is – please fix it." Whether you actually vocalize it or not, your approach should be, "I have this pain problem. What can you *and I* do about it?"

The patient has to take the basic responsibility?

That's right. It all comes back to the very first point I made in Chapter 1. A lot of it has to do with developing a positive attitude. If you're consciously trying to get well, you stand a far better chance of succeeding than if you just sit back and say, "Make me recover." That's true of virtually any ailment, but it's especially important when part of the problem is psychological or emotional, as it so often is with chronic pain. You will not help yourself by assuming a passive role and, by default, learning to be disabled. I can't overemphasize the value of attempting to take control, thinking of yourself as a recovering person, even if you suffer some setbacks, and working actively to succeed with the treatment your doctor prescribes.

Early in the consultation, you and your doctor should agree on a goal, such as reducing your pain or, even more important, getting you back to work.

And while setting a goal, you should get a realistic estimate of how long the treatment should take to produce the desired results. With chronic pain, you need patience. You can't expect to be rid of your problem in a matter of days; it's bound to take weeks or even months – but not forever. Whoever helps you set your goal should also help you fix a reasonable timetable for reaching it.

Finally, if your problem is definitely the chronic pain syndrome, your doctor may arrange for you to visit a pain clinic for help from a specially trained team of doctors, psychologists, physical therapists, and social workers. These specialists will try to help you by prescribing appropriate action or treatment while carefully monitoring and recording your progress. If you are afflicted by CPS, or headed in that direction, you will be encouraged to alter your pattern of living, so that you see the problem in a new light and can take charge, once again, of the decision-making process, rather than allowing your pain to dictate the decisions you make.

Does this sort of professional help work better if I'm part of a group?

Yes, often that is an important factor, just as it is for people who are struggling with alcoholism or drug addiction.

At one pain clinic, in Miami, patients are encouraged to make a contest out of breaking the medication habit. Each patient's pill consumption becomes a matter of daily record known to the whole class: "Mr. Green took seven pills today; Mrs. White took five. . . ." Patients who manage to reduce their dosages are rewarded by a healthy sense of accomplishment and praise from their peers.

Many clinics help patients kick their drug habits by making pill-taking time-dependent, rather than pain-dependent. That is, a person isn't allowed a pill because he has pain; he's given a pill at a specified time, regardless of his pain. The patient soon learns he can't "earn" a pill by feeling pain. He has to wait until the appointed hour. The association between pain and pill-taking is thereby disrupted while the intervals between doses are gradually extended, to taper off consumption.

Do most patients who have gone through that routine learn to get along without medication?

Not as often as everyone would like. But you have to realize that apart from dependence on pills, pain itself is addictive, and giving it up can be as tough as giving up smoking, drinking, and sex – all at the same time.

You also have to allow for the fact that chronic pain clinics are bound to have a high rate of failure, because they take on the worst cases, including some incurables – people who have lived with the syndrome for too long. People like that reach a point where they don't just tolerate their pain but envelop themselves in it until it becomes virtually inescapable. Pain clinics face greater challenges than those my colleagues and I face in the classes we conduct for back patients. While our classes can often succeed by dispensing an ounce of prevention, the pain clinics have to offer a pound of cure – and, often, even a pound is not nearly enough.

As I mentioned earlier, people suffering from continual pain can become particularly self-centered and demanding, and many of them will not put up with the rigid rules and schedules that are necessary features of most pain clinics. If you check into one of these clinics, you will be told you must get up every morning at eight o'clock, pain or no pain, eat breakfast at eight-thirty, go out for a walk at nine, and so on. . . .

You aren't allowed to decide, "I won't go out for my walk today because my pain feels worse." Pain or no pain, you take that walk on schedule. The whole idea of such discipline is to reintroduce the patient to habits that bear no reference to pain. But some patients can't stick to that routine for long because it doesn't fit the pattern they have developed to suit their pain, and they soon drop out of the program.

Would such people stand a better chance with a psychiatrist?

Possibly, although the prospects are not as good as you might suppose. Some fine work has been done in this field lately by certain psychiatrists who have taken a special interest in pain. But psychiatrists on the whole have not had much success in treating the chronic pain syndrome. Without some special training or background in pain therapy, a psychiatrist may not appreciate how the patient's pain response works as part of a closed loop, with pain producing muscle tension, and muscle tension producing pain, and both factors being magnified by fear and other emotions. Often, the psychiatrist will focus on extrinsic factors such as sexual hangups, job dissatisfaction, and stress in the family – problems that are actually byproducts of the pain – without touching on the underlying cause. For this reason, many pain treatment programs use psychologists instead because of their greater emphasis on behavior modification.

Even if the psychiatrist succeeds in helping solve those extrinsic problems, the patient will still have the original minor back trouble, and, more important, the chronic pain syndrome it produced. At this point the psychiatrist, aware of the patient's back trouble, is likely to announce: "Your problem is not in your head; you need to see an orthopedic surgeon." The surgeon, finding no back condition severe enough to account for the patient's pain, and recognizing the exaggeration of symptoms during the physical examination, will probably declare: "There's nothing wrong with your back; you should see a psychiatrist."

At any rate, most pain patients are reluctant to see psychiatrists because of the implication that the pain must be a sign of mental illness. What these people need is someone who not only understands pain but also has the ability to guide them through the process of behavior modification; someone who can explain that the problem is not a mental disorder and then provide appropriate physical treatment. It matters little whether they choose a surgeon, a psychiatrist, a psychologist, or a family physician, as long as it's a professional who has had experience with the syndrome and can appreciate the difficulties of helping its sufferers re-order their habits and responses into an entirely new lifestyle.

What sort of difficulties does a person face in trying to break out of the syndrome?

We have touched on some of them already: dependence on medication, for instance. Resolving that problem will mean eliminating the use of pills completely or at least finding ways of controlling the habit, so as to avoid abuse.

Drugs, by the way, are often partly to blame for the personality changes that occur in many chronic pain victims. In retrospect, I feel that was so in my own case, during my time in Scotland. I was taking so many narcotics that I began looking forward to the pleasant floating sensation that followed every dose. Finally, I concluded I could be subconsciously nurturing my pain to justify taking the pills. I said to myself, "This is becoming a very bad loop" – and I quit the medication.

Partly because of that experience, perhaps, I am not so quick to condemn chronic pain patients who misuse their drugs.

Does the desire for medication inevitably develop into out-and-out addiction?

For some people, drug overuse for chronic pain is a route to addiction. But I know many patients who can take a high dose of pain killers day after day, without ever increasing it. While they are dependent, they do not abuse the drugs as most addicts do.

One patient of mine, after six back operations, still suffers chronic pain, for which she takes five aspirin-codeine pills a day. That means she is getting a hefty dose of both drugs. No question about it, this woman is hooked on those pills; but she doesn't abuse them. Even after a recent fall down stairs, which shook her up pretty badly, and no doubt increased her pain, she did not increase her dosage but stuck to those five pills a day.

Certainly I hope she will start decreasing her dosage. Her family doctor has threatened to cut off her prescription; he keeps telling her those pills are not good for her. He's right, of course. But should he cut off the prescription? Here we have a woman who has undergone many surgical procedures, mostly attempted fusions and refusions. By now she has enough scar tissue in her spine to give her all the pain she'll ever need. Yet, with the help of those pills, she's living with her situation. She is a successful sales representative, with one of the best records in the whole company.

I'm afraid of what will happen if her pills are suddenly cut off. She'll adopt more blatant pain behavior: she'll take to her bed, give up her job and income, and become a totally depressed individual.

I have encouraged her to cut down – even reducing her intake to four pills a day would be a real accomplishment – and I have outlined a scheme for her to follow. But meanwhile, in the choice between the two extremes, she has picked what I consider the lesser of two evils.

Is overcoming drug dependence the main problem, then, in escaping the pain syndrome?

No, there are usually several other important problems to solve. For example, some patients become dependent on their physical treatments.

How can physical treatments become habit-forming?

Many physical treatments are forms of passive therapy where the patient is not required to expend any effort or take any responsibility. Someone or something else reduces the pain and makes the patient feel better. Passive treatment from a physical therapist, chiropractor, or massage therapist can produce great temporary relief. But without a change in the patient's behavior, the pain is certain to return. So the therapy becomes the only source of hope.

But at least it gives the person some hope. On that basis, taking the physical treatment sounds perfectly logical to me.

Oh, it's logical enough. But in order to get well, you must not become heavily dependent on *any* outside help. If you do, you'll create a self-fulfilling prophecy. It's fine to believe your physical treatments can help you. But it's not healthy to believe you can't get along without them. If you are going to get well, you must believe most of all in yourself – in your ability to take charge and bring about your own recovery. Your pain may not be "all in your head" but the ability to conquer that pain *has* to be in *your* head – or it's nowhere.

When a patient asks me, "Should I go back for more physical therapy?" I have to weigh the alternatives: will more short-term management benefit this patient or merely create or reinforce an unwanted dependency?

My decision will depend partly on whether I think the patient is being positive or negative. I will approve the therapy if I believe the question means, "I want to help myself by means of more physical therapy," but not if it seems to mean, "I don't know what to do – I think I'll let someone else take away my pain."

Self-assurance is obviously the key.

It's essential, all right, but gaining self-assurance is not easy; and it may be especially difficult if legal considerations are complicating the medical and emotional situation. That can happen to accident victims who get into litigation over damages.

How does the prospect of litigation work against a pain patient?

Several ways. Early in a dispute over an injury, a lawyer will customarily obtain a doctor's report and turn a copy over to his client, the patient. We've already seen how Doctor can make an injury sound worse than it actually is, and a medical report written as part of a legal claim can make scary reading. If it supports your case, it's also likely to support your pain – and perhaps aggravate it by making you fearful that you will never recover.

Unfortunately, the legal process can drag on and on, as we all know, and as long as your lawsuit is pending, you have an unhealthy incentive to keep right on feeling pain. Especially if your lawyer calls up and says, "How's your sore back? Don't forget we go to court again tomorrow."

Just the other day, a patient made a remark to me that unfortunately is all too typical. She's a woman who suffered a neck injury in a rear-end collision about a year and a half ago. On previous visits she had told me her pain was gradually subsiding. Then, on this last occasion, she said: "I'd almost forgotten about my neck pain, but my lawyer told me to come back and see you to be re-assessed. And so I started thinking about my pain again, and it came back."

You can hardly blame the lawyer for wanting an up-to-date medical opinion of his client's condition, but there's no doubt in my mind that many accident victims would recover faster if there were no such things as legal claims and lawsuits. According to some studies, people who resort to litigation over injuries seldom get better until their lawsuits are settled.

Certainly I am convinced that for the patient's sake a case should be settled as quickly as possible. I've seen too many instances where prolonged litigation or an insurance investigation has led to the development of chronic pain problems that remained long after the back injury itself had healed.

The negative effects of litigation on a patient's recovery have been observed by specialists who have studied the problem more systematically than I have. In an article they co-wrote for an insurance journal, a lawyer and psychologist cautioned that "... plaintiff counsel should not simply push ahead with the lawsuit without regard to the effect that this has on his client. He should never be unmindful of the fact that it is just as important, if not more important, for his client to get better as ... to get compensated."*

Another pain specialist has even coined an expression, "nomogenic illness," to denote the condition brought about or contributed to by lawyers and the legal process.**

If you're embarking on a lawsuit, that's a hazard you ought to be aware of.

Does it follow, then, that patients improve dramatically as soon as their lawsuits are settled?

Unfortunately, no. Various studies on this issue have produced contradictory statistics. In one study, all but 10 percent of patients involved in litigation got better as soon as their legal cases were settled. In other studies, as many as 50 percent failed to get better even after receiving settlements.

What do you think held their recovery back at that point?

We can only speculate, but I think one reason is that money is poor compensation for what the injury has done to disrupt, if not destroy, their lives. More important, because of the duration of their symptoms, many of these people have accepted their new invalid lifestyle as permanent. Partly because of the image pre-

---

*Crawford M. MacIntyre, QC, and Dr. David T. Corey, MA, PhD, in "The Chronic Pain Syndrome," published in *Without Prejudice*, November 1983.

**Dr. Milo Tyndel, Toronto psychiatrist and neurologist, cited by MacIntyre and Corey in "The Chronic Pain Syndrome."

sented in court, they see themselves as disabled persons con-
demned to a life of pain. Any form of physical or emotional stress,
no matter how commonplace, is related in their minds to the
accident. The resultant muscle tension triggers a typical attack
of pain. They have developed a learned response that is beyond
their control.

**Can you offer a few guidelines for people with chronic pain who
want to avoid becoming trapped in the syndrome?**

Yes. The first step is to get a complete and accurate diagnosis.
That means finding a doctor who will listen to your needs, provide
moral support, and eliminate any doubts you may have about
serious physical problems. You can't hope to conquer your pain
if you keep worrying about what's "really" wrong.

Next, you have to resolve to take charge of your situation, and
not delude yourself that you are coping with the problem when
you simply avoid painful activities. It helps if you refuse to accept
the pain as part of yourself but look at it instead as an adversary
that you can struggle against – and overcome. And the truth is
that you *can* overcome the pain if you *believe* you can.

The third step is to profit from mistakes other people have
made in your situation. It's a common mistake to give in to the
pain by becoming completely inactive. The doctor tells you, "Be
careful not to over-exert yourself," and so you do nothing but
sit around and vegetate. After a week or two, you can't stand the
inactivity, and so you rush out and spend a whole day gardening
or playing golf. Next day, not surprisingly, your muscles feel sore
all over. Worse than that, you feel guilty because you didn't follow
the doctor's advice. And so you take yourself off to bed, resolving
not even to tell the doctor what you've done. That's a common
cycle for CPS patients: frustration leading to over-exertion leading
to more pain and frustration.

**What's a better course of action if you're told not to over-exert
yourself?**

Practice moderation – moderate exercise, as prescribed by your
doctor, and moderation in your daily activities. And be prepared
to tolerate some pain. Keep in mind that if you have just gone

through a period of inactivity, you should ease gradually back into your regular routine – a little each day until your muscles begin to recover their normal tone. Don't forget that simple muscular soreness is not indicative of a serious problem. And gentle exercise, even with chronic pain, won't cause any harm.

You are bound to have moments of doubt, particularly when you try slightly more strenuous activities and you find that the pain increases. You'll be inclined to wonder, "My god, what am I doing to myself?" This is a crucial point in your recovery when, with support from an understanding doctor or therapist, you need to muster all the self-confidence you can. You must appreciate that if you carry on now and put up with the pain, you will be rewarded by some real progress.

But if you give in to the pain and reduce your activity, you will fall into a destructive downward spiral. A decrease in your activity will cause your pain to subside, and you'll probably spend five or six weeks resting while telling yourself you're doing the only safe and sane thing. In fact you are not really solving the problem at all and could even be making your next attempt more difficult.

Sooner or later, possibly at your doctor's urging, you will try to get up and around again. This time, the pain will be much more immediate – much harder to take. The reason, although you may not realize it, will be both physical and psychological: after weeks of inactivity, your muscles are sure to hurt. And the moment you feel the discomfort, you will tell yourself, "There it is! I knew it would happen! My pain is back!"

Like an animal in some psychologist's experiment, you have developed a conditioned response. You have learned that activity means pain, and so you avoid activity. And each time you try and fail, you reinforce that conditioning.

Probably without realizing it, you are establishing a pattern of behavior that is carrying you to the brink of the chronic pain syndrome.

To avoid that pattern, you must recognize that if you've been inactive, muscular pain is inevitable but not intolerable. And it will not persist, once those muscles become properly conditioned again. Imagine putting your normal elbow in a cast for six weeks. When you first try to move your arm again, you'll feel a great deal of pain from simple joint stiffness and weak muscles. The proper treatment, of course, would be to start active movement in spite of the discomfort. How much more trouble would you have if you treated the pain by putting your elbow back in the cast for another six weeks?

You should realize that if you fall into the habit of saying, "Every time I do such and such, I get pain," then you certainly *will* get pain. Instead, tell yourself, "I know such and such activity won't actually harm me, and so I am going to do it whether it hurts or not."

That's an important step towards dissociating normal activity from pain. If you can do that, you will achieve what the best pain clinics try to do. Their objective, stated broadly, is to "normalize" the person's behavior by shifting his or her responses from a pain-dominated lifestyle to an activity-dominated lifestyle.

In one pain clinic, for instance, the therapists require patients to walk a specific distance every day, regardless of the pain. Each day's walk is timed and the time is recorded. On the first day, the person can take virtually all the time he wants, but he is encouraged to improve on that time during each subsequent walk. Typically, a patient will keep improving the pace without realizing it, until the records are brought out as proof. As the improvement continues, patients find themselves concentrating more on the achievement than on the pain, and gradually they come to realize that pain is not an inevitable result of walking.

If a person has felt crippled for some time, that discovery must seem like a great revelation.

It is – it's an immense source of satisfaction, not only because it shows progress but also because activity in itself is a satisfying thing. Which brings me to my final point of these guidelines: the best way to get back to normal is to start acting as though you *are* normal.

Patients say to me, "I can't go back to work – I'm still having pain." And I always say, "Don't tell anybody. Just go back to work and put up with a little pain." I point out that working regularly is far less risky than remaining idle, trying to wait out the pain and playing the role of a disabled person. I get quite frustrated and occasionally furious when a patient of mine is ready to return to work but is prevented from doing so by his company or union because he is not considered fully recovered. It's often hard to make the powers that be understand that getting back on the job is an essential part of getting better. Forcing a person to remain inactive is unnecessary and potentially destructive.

And so my advice is: *get active as soon as possible, even if it hurts a little.* How does that old expression go – "Short-term pain for long-term gain"?

Believe me, if it steers you clear of the chronic pain syndrome, it's well worth the discomfort.

7. INTERCOURSE, PREGNANCY, AND YOUR PAINFUL BACK

In my view, the impact of back pain on your sex life has to be seen in the wide context of all your living habits. Too often, when we talk about sex we speak of it as though it were entirely isolated from the rest of our experience. We forget that in sexual relations, back problems create the same cycles of fear and pain – and the same opportunities to control situations – as in other aspects of everyday living.

Sometimes, too, you may find it easier to dwell on your back pain than to work at improving your sex life. I'm not a marriage counselor, and this book can't cover all the ramifications of a sexual relationship that has a back problem as one of its ingredients. But what I have heard from a great many patients convinces me that even though back pain is real, it too often serves merely as an excuse for inadequate sexual response.

If that observation hits home, you should understand that severe back pain does not necessarily indicate a severe physical problem, that your backache can become a serious sexual problem only if you allow it to do so.

What are the hazards of having sexual intercourse if you suffer chronic back pain?

The greatest hazard lies in letting your bad back interfere with your sex life. Allowing that to happen can ruin the whole relationship.

But surely the activity involved in intercourse can be harmful in some cases.

Almost never. It may cause pain but it won't cause damage. Mind you, the fear of pain is genuine, and some people with bad backs truly believe they are going to harm themselves during the excitement of intercourse – but they won't.

You can't hurt your back that way?

No – for two reasons. First, while strenuous exertion might rarely be harmful during a brief attack of acute back pain, the danger doesn't arise, because you're not likely to feel sexy when your back is killing you.

Second, as I can't stress often enough, there's a world of difference between *hurt* and *harm*. There are a thousand things you can do to various parts of your body that will hurt temporarily without harming you. Standing on one leg for half an hour would probably hurt quite a lot but it wouldn't do you any harm. Having sex when your back is not at its best may hurt a little – it may even take the joy out of sex on that one occasion – but it's not going to harm you – or your back. On the other hand, however, great harm could come from denying yourself the opportunity for intimacy and depriving your partner of pleasure and gratification. Whenever I hear of people avoiding sex because of a bad back, I'm concerned there is something else wrong with their relationship. Without either partner being aware of it, the back pain may have become the excuse for saying no. Otherwise, the person with the back problem would say, "Let's try. Even if it hurts a little, it'll still be worth it!"

So the situation calls for a certain amount of positive thinking?

Definitely. Otherwise, it's like being a prizefighter and stepping into the ring with an opponent you know is going to beat you. If that's your attitude, you're sure to lose. If you believe your back condition will defeat you, it will. But if you take the opposite attitude, you'll come out a winner.

Obviously there's a big emotional factor at work.

No question about it. What starts out as one person's relatively simple physical problem can soon cause both partners to get bogged down in a morass of emotions – fear, inadequacy, resentment, recrimination, and guilt. And once these emotions appear, they feed on one another.

Which partner feels guilty – the one with the sore back?

Sooner or later, they both do. Usually, they feel a mixture of emotions. The backache sufferer either feels guilty for refusing to have sex or feels resentful or inadequate when they do have it. The partner feels guilty for pursuing the idea when the other person obviously doesn't want to, or feels resentful or rejected because their sex life has disappeared. Those negative emotions just keep bouncing back and forth. Pretty soon the back-pain-versus-sex issue dominates their whole relationship.

But what if one person says quite honestly, "I can't have sex because my back hurts?"

In some cases, for a short while, that may be perfectly true. But often it needn't be. It *becomes* true because of the way people respond to the idea. It's another self-fulfilling prophecy.

Picture it: two people go to bed ostensibly with a delightful purpose in mind. But they are all too aware that one of them has a back problem. Instead of saying, "Let's find a way to make love in spite of it," they just lie there asking, "But what about your [my] back?"

What chance do two people have of being happy and successful lovers when they're worrying about a worn facet joint or a ruptured disc? After a while, they're talking like people in a medical clinic instead of lovers in a bedroom. Obviously, the romantic mood is shattered. And that's the simpler scenario. It gets a lot more complicated when one partner begins using back pain as an excuse for avoiding sex.

The back sufferer's equivalent of "Not tonight, darling, I have a headache"?

Exactly. It can – and does – mask an enormous number of problems in relationships. I can think of many instances where patients of mine have gone to great lengths to point out that it wasn't the emotional side of their relationship but only the back pain that was preventing them from having intercourse. In most cases I got the feeling that these people were protesting just a little too much.

Are most back specialists conscious of this emotional factor affecting their patients' sex lives?

Oh, I'm sure they realize the potential is there. But the physical aspects of a back assessment are extensive, and it's easy for a doctor to focus on them, to the exclusion of other aspects.

Also, back examinations are seldom carried out in what you might describe as a counseling environment. For example, I see many of my patients in a clinic – a big room with cubicles where conversations are easily overheard. While my patients don't seem to mind if someone else hears them telling me about their back pains, they are not about to broach the subject of sex.

Shouldn't doctors ask patients whether their sex life is being impaired by their backache?

Many of us do – if we have any inkling there's a problem. But even when we see patients who present us with sexual problems, we haven't the time or the facilities – or for that matter the training – to provide the necessary counseling.

Then what do you do about it?

I hear the patient out and make whatever comments I think might be helpful, and then I usually refer him or her to a psychologist or other counselor. Before I recommend a referral, however, I make sure the patient understands that the problem is real and physical and that I am not suggesting for a moment that it's all in their head. I consider that important because I have found that many patients otherwise resent having a surgeon refer them to someone for psychological consultation.

Do you think many of your patients have back-related sex problems they never discuss with you?

Yes, I'm sure of it. I also suspect there are those who don't even realize that a sexual problem can originate with backache. I'm always glad when a patient confides in me, and I do what I can to provide some preliminary guidance or support.

At one of my clinics recently, I was conducting an examination on a woman who has been a patient of mine for about ten years. Still in her thirties, she had been married for the second time about six months earlier, and she brought her new husband to the clinic with her.

I had finished examining her and was giving her my assessment when she asked if she and her husband could talk to me privately. Of course I agreed, and so we found a quiet office away from the other patients and staff. As soon as the three of us were alone, I began to understand the real reason why the woman had come to the clinic that day.

She was quite frank about their situation. It seems that she and her new husband had had an excellent sexual relationship before they were married, but now they were having serious problems. Her back pain was interfering with their sex life. She couldn't lie on her back. It hurt her to place her legs in the right position. It hurt her to raise her hips up. She just couldn't perform sexually. It was all too painful. And she was really frightened that the marriage would falter because her husband wasn't able to get sexual satisfaction.

If she hadn't asked for that private conversation, I would have done the assessment and prescribed treatment – mainly exercise in her case – without realizing that the main issue was not her back pain but her sexual relationship with her husband.

What could you – or did you – do for her?

We talked about things they could do to relieve the problem, or at least get around it. Oral sex was one thing. Some people have inhibitions about oral sex, but it can be a gentle yet stimulating aid to good sexual relations. It can be especially useful in foreplay, to achieve arousal without the kind of physical exertion that so often aggravates back pain.

We also talked about various positions for intercourse that would avoid back pain or at least reduce it to a tolerable level.

Are there certain positions that are generally better for most back patients?

Yes, but it's often a matter of trial and error, and the best solution will often depend on which partner has back pain. For instance, if the woman has Type One back pain, the so-called missionary position, with the man on top, may hurt, since it requires the woman to lie on her back, causing her spine to arch. She can help the situation by keeping both knees bent, but the movements necessary for intercourse may still jar the spinal joints and produce discomfort. Instead, the couple might exchange positions, to have the woman lying on top, supporting her upper torso with her arms and resting on her knees to keep her back bent forward slightly.

Another good possibility is the spoon position, with both partners on their sides, both facing in the same direction, with their legs bent and the woman in front and slightly higher up on the bed than the man, so that he can enter from behind.

If the woman has pain originating in a disc, she may find she is comfortable on her hands and knees, so that rear entry is possible without a great deal of movement on her part.

It's possible, too, to help a woman with backache achieve sexual union even if she finds it painful to part her legs. If she lies on her back, with her legs together but with the knees slightly bent, her partner can spread his legs to straddle her. Or if she lies face down, again with her legs slightly bent, her partner will be able to gain at least a limited degree of penetration – more than you might expect. It's not an ideal way to go about it, but it can produce satisfactory results for both partners.

What about the missionary position when the man is the one with back pain?

He won't care for that position either if he has a facet problem, since it will be painful for him to arch his back. But he can improve matters by supporting his upper body with his arms and keeping his back flexed forward.

Are there any basic rules?

Not really. Try to choose a position that calls for a movement other than the one that hurts. In the missionary position, either partner may aggravate Type One pain unless he or she takes special care. In contrast, Type Two symptoms can be made worse with forward thrusting of the pelvis, a movement much like the pelvic tilt, which increases disc pressure. I know that many couples find it satisfactory for the man to lie on his back while the woman sits with her knees astride his body, using her arms or elbows to support her upper body. She may be face to face with him or facing toward his feet – whichever is preferable.

It sounds as though some couples might have to depart from their customary style.

That's right. But that can be good for any long-term relationship. In addition, a lot of people, especially after they have been together for a number of years, tend to overlook the importance of extensive foreplay. With very little foreplay, intercourse itself may involve an excessive amount of movement for both partners to reach orgasm. With prolonged foreplay, that final period of activity can probably be much shorter and less strenuous – to the benefit of the partner with backache.

Are some positions wrong for anyone with back trouble?

Yes, some positions are obviously hard on the back, and you will steer clear of them almost automatically. And if you have discovered during some other routine activity that a certain posture or stance is painful you wouldn't even consider it for intercourse.

What positions are likely to be a problem?

One obvious example, for a man with a bad back, is the standing position, where he holds his partner in his arms with her legs around his body. That's a macho stance that could strain even a healthy back.

Bending forward with the knees straight will often increase discogenic back pain – as you may have discovered in other situations – and it certainly should be avoided during lovemaking. The same can be said of any position that causes excessive arching of the back, since it can bring on pain from the spinal joints; the idea is to find a neutral or stress-free posture.

If the woman has Type One backache, she'll probably want to avoid lying, face down, over the edge of the bed, if her legs dangle free. This lack of support will require her to arch her back to maintain the position, causing stress on the small facet joints.

Similarly, if she lies on her back with her legs draped over the edge of the bed and her feet unsupported, she will automatically arch her back. She won't be able to bend her knees, and she may not have enough strength in her abdominal muscles alone to maintain a pelvic tilt and avoid the back pain. The moral, I guess, is that even if the romance of the moment has your head in the clouds, it's a good idea to keep your feet on the ground.

Incidentally, that last position is fine for a couple where the woman has no spinal problems and the man is the one with the sore back.

What would your general advice be?

The best general advice can be summed up in a word: experiment. Of course, we have to hope that the couple are able to voice their needs and desires in an open and positive way, so that nobody is fumbling around in the dark, so to speak, surprising the other person with variations that haven't been discussed and that may prove unpleasant or painful.

If you have some reservations about positions you might try, but are not confident that they will help you avoid back pain, try them out some time when you're alone. Simulate intercourse without your partner, to get a better idea whether the positions you have in mind will be comfortable.

Would it be worthwhile to get a book showing various sexual positions?

By all means. Explore the possibilities and try anything that might please you and your partner. Just remember that whatever keeps your back from hurting, and makes the rest of you feel good, is all right. There are no absolutes. Mind you, if you show up in the bedroom one night with an ironing board, a block and tackle, and a set of shoulder straps, you might not receive the response you were hoping for, no matter how good it might make your back feel.

What about sexual activity following surgery? Do you have any special rules for that?

That depends. If there are bones that need time to fuse, or stitches that might pull out, you obviously shouldn't exert yourself in any way without your doctor's approval. Other than that, the principle is the same as for other times when your back is a problem: as long as you have a gentle and considerate partner, let your inclinations be your guide.

That point is made in an old gag that some back doctors still use. The patient asks: "How soon after the operation can I have sex?" and the doctor replies, "That depends on whether you have a private or semi-private room." In other words, if you have the urge for sex, you are well enough to enjoy it – harmlessly.

Apart from potential pain during intercourse, do back problems affect people's sexual capacity in any way?

Some men with back pain find it impossible to achieve an erection, but this problem is fairly rare.

Why can't they achieve an erection?

In most cases, it's psychological. We're not talking about getting an erection during an actual attack of back pain. As I've already pointed out, hardly anybody feels sexy at a time like that.

However, even during a pain-free period, a man with chronic backache may have a psychological block that inhibits him from having an erection. He may fear that intercourse will bring on pain that can paralyze him, although that actually never happens. It's as fanciful as the time-worn story of the passionate couple who are making love when the man has a back spasm and is so paralyzed he can't withdraw. He and his lady friend, unable to separate, have to be carried away on a stretcher. In the more imaginative accounts, the whole thing happens at high noon in Times Square, while thousands of amused spectators look on. That's all sheer nonsense, of course. A spasm could interrupt a person's sexual activity but certainly not cause paralysis. The worst that happens is that a man's fear of back pain makes him impotent.

Could his failure to achieve an erection be physical rather than psychological?

Yes – although physical causes are even more rare, and of course they are not necessarily related to a back problem. One physical problem is an insufficient supply of blood, which can be due to hardening or blockage of some arteries. Another physical cause is neurological, involving nerve damage that may interfere with normal sexual function. But again, let me emphasize that compared to psychological causes, physical factors are a far less common reason for failure to achieve an erection.

Whatever the cause may be, failure to achieve an erection must be a frightening experience.

Impotence does scare a lot of men. But there is really no need to be frightened about back pain preventing an erection. It helps a man immensely to realize it's usually a temporary psychological condition that can be remedied. Otherwise, it may become self-perpetuating. If a man is afraid he can't have an erection, there's a strong chance he won't be able to. But once he knows that other men have had the same experience and have recovered easily, he can keep his back pain in perspective.

So you could almost invoke the old expression about having nothing to fear but fear itself.

As far as the actual impotence goes, that's quite true. I suspect a lot of men harbor these fears and experience impotence because, for whatever reason, they never discuss the problem with a doctor or other professional counselor.

For the same reason other sexual problems don't get discussed with doctors?

That's probably part of the answer. Not many men are likely to bring up the subject, and some doctors may see no way of broaching it without embarrassing their patients. Which is another way of saying the doctor hasn't developed his consultative techniques very well.

Or a doctor may ask questions the wrong way. "How's your sex life?" is practically an invitation for the patient to answer, "Fine." A lot of men would find it demeaning to admit otherwise. The doctor would likely get a more revealing answer if he were to say, "A lot of men with your kind of back trouble find it difficult to get an erection. It's frightening, but it can usually be corrected very easily. If you ever have a problem that way, let's talk about it." I think most men will respond frankly to that sort of approach – and a great many cases that have remained secret can be recognized and dealt with.

How does a doctor deal with impotence?

The first step, obviously, is to determine the cause – whether the problem is related to the man's back condition or to some other problem. The doctor can test for the physical reasons: that is, poor blood supply or nerve damage. If there is no physical cause, it's probably a psychological issue, and the next step is to refer the patient for counseling.

Women obviously have their own reasons to be concerned about back problems. For instance, what about menstruation as a cause of back pain?

Although some of the pain occurring during menstruation is felt in the lower back, it's different from common backache. It has to do with muscle spasms in the uterus, which occur as the result of changes in the hormone levels. Fortunately, there are now medications that can provide effective relief.

Menstruation can also cause fluid accumulation throughout the body. This leads to swelling in the tissues, including the tissues in the back. And if the woman already has sore back muscles, the added fluid – the edema – will increase their irritability and aggravate the problems that already bother her spine.

Backache is something many women fear when they consider having a baby. Is it true that pregnant women inevitably get back pain?

Not inevitably, no. And if backache is going to show up at all, it usually does so around the fourth or fifth month of the pregnancy and often disappears again by the end of the seventh month. Of course most pregnant women do feel some back pain right before delivery. I think it helps to realize that pregnancy doesn't usually initiate the problem of back pain; all it does is add temporary stress to the back.

What about a woman who has had back pain in the past? Is she certain to have back pain during pregnancy?

Not necessarily. I've seen some women with a history of back pain who went through pregnancy with no increase in their problem, or even with no back pain at all. I've seen other women whose initial attack of back pain developed as the result of a normal pregnancy. With many women, pregnancy brought them their first bout with back pain because it imposed extra strain on a back that had already become worn from normal use. Sometimes a woman will get backache for the first time while bearing her third or fourth child. It wouldn't be accurate to say her back pain was caused by that last pregnancy; all her pregnancies contributed something to the strain. My favorite analogy is the frayed rope on an old-fashioned backyard swing. Year after year, the rope encircling the tree branch becomes more and more frayed. Then, one day, some boy who's too heavy for the swing jumps on and starts pumping. Of course the rope, which is almost frayed through by now, breaks. You can't really say the rope broke because that one boy used the swing. It broke because it was worn and couldn't take the extra strain.

Then getting pregnant does entail some risk to your back?

That depends what you mean by risk. Certainly there is a possibility that back pain will develop; I suppose it's risky in that sense. But there is no danger to either mother or child from the back pain that occurs in pregnancy.

Are the causes of a pregnant woman's back pain the same as the causes of common backache?

In most cases, yes, although pregnancy may add some special stresses of its own. Even before her pregnancy is obvious to the casual observer, a woman may adopt a characteristic gait that is different from her normal walk. She leans back a little; her toes point outward, with a gait that is an unmistakable sign of her condition.

This change in her walk places unaccustomed strain on certain muscles. Her body begins releasing hormones that will relax the ligaments of her pelvis, so that it can stretch open at the time of birth. Once the ligaments have become more lax, she is more vulnerable to an attack of back pain, specifically from the joints in the back of the pelvis, at the base of the spine.

Also, in the later stages of pregnancy, the weight of the unborn baby strains the mother's back and abdominal muscles in much the same way that a fat man's pot belly puts extra strain on his spine.

All these conditions contribute to back pain. Occasionally the primary location of the pain is in the sacroiliac joint – where the spine connects with the back of the pelvis. But the distinction is rather academic since ordinary low-back pain, though starting a little further up the spine, will usually radiate into the same area. To a woman with a chronic back complaint who has lately become pregnant, it seems like the same old pain. Even her doctor will probably find it hard to decide where the pain originates. But it really doesn't make much difference. The problem is the same, simple wear and tear. For all practical purposes, if pregnancy-related back pain does occur, it should be regarded as just another episode of common backache – and treated accordingly.

Perhaps the most difficult situation arises when a pregnant woman develops Type Three back pain – that is, the uncommon variety where a nerve is actually pinched. A case of this kind can be a real challenge for any doctor to manage. Chemical injection is out of the question because of the risk it presents to the baby, and I would rule out surgery as well, except in maybe one case in a thousand where the indications for surgery were overwhelming. Fortunately, most of the cases of nerve-root pressure get better, given time, rest, and the various other remedies that assist recovery whether someone is pregnant or not.

Aren't there any specific forms of back pain that are caused by pregnancy?

Yes, there are a few that arise because of the position of the baby, and there are others related to the complications that may arise from the pregnancy. In this case, however, the back pain is always secondary to other symptoms that the family physician or obstetrician will recognize as being related directly to pregnancy. Simple back pain in the absence of any other complaints can be pretty uncomfortable, but it is harmless.

You may have heard the term "back labor." Some women in labor experience a back pain that is different from common backache. The pain is quite low, often in the flanks. It's a form of pain that is part of normal delivery – although in a slightly unusual location. While it can be very unpleasant, it is just related to the intense muscular activity of the uterus at the time of birth and does not lead to long-term problems or increase the incidence of future episodes of back pain.

Are there some women whose backs are in such bad shape that they simply should not even consider getting pregnant?

Absolutely not. I've had patients tell me they have been given that advice, and I think it's wrong. Pregnancy could increase the expectant mother's back pain, but none of the mechanical problems that affect people's backs make pregnancy dangerous or impossible.

This was not always true. At one time, the spinal condition called spondylolisthesis was a threat to some pregnant women. Spondylolisthesis is not a disease but a mechanical disorder in which one vertebra slips out of line. It was identified for the first time more than a century ago as the cause of one woman's inability to deliver normally. In her case the slippage at the lowest level of the lumbar spine was so bad that her spinal column had moved forward into her pelvis and blocked the birth canal.

But before you start worrying about that possibility, let me emphasize two points. That degree of spondylolisthesis is extremely rare, but even if it occurs it can now be identified easily on X-ray and corrected with current surgical techniques. Also, if that severe slip does occur and is still undiagnosed when the patient becomes pregnant, it can be detected early in labor, and the baby can be delivered safely by Caesarean section.

What do you recommend for women with back pain who are going to have babies?

Exercise and special habits in daily living are important – but not just for women with a history of back pain. Every woman should exercise during and after pregnancy, to reduce the unwanted effects of child-bearing and promote a speedy return to normal activity once the baby is born.

What sorts of exercises?

When she first sees her family doctor or obstetrician about her pregnancy, she will probably be told to take up certain exercises that are commonly prescribed for expectant mothers. They are intended to strengthen the muscles of the abdomen and the pelvic floor. This helps support the unborn baby and will eventually assist with the delivery. This exercise program is similar in many ways to the one I prescribe for Type One back pain but, as with any set of exercises, experimentation is important. The expectant mother should develop a program that fits her daily routine and works to minimize her discomfort.

Are there special exercises for women whose pain is originating in the sacroiliac joint?

Yes, but special sacroiliac joint exercises are rarely necessary. Most expectant mothers find that regular back exercises provide the pain relief they are looking for.

What special habits should the pregnant woman adopt for daily living?

Various tricks can spare her back from unnecessary strain:

- She probably won't need to be told to leave her high heels in the closet and get herself some flat shoes. She'll discover that high heels increase the lordosis or curve in her lower spine, pushing the mid-section further forward and increasing the mechanical strain.
- She should make use of a foot-rest while seated, whenever possible, since this will take the strain off her back by raising her legs and reducing any excessive curve in her spine. Resting with the feet in an elevated position helps support the weight of the abdomen. It's useful as well because keeping the feet up will reduce swelling in the legs and aching in the thigh muscles.
- Rest is important too, of course. A pregnant woman will find she needs plenty of sleep each night, and she should take daytime naps as well, if possible.

How soon should a new mother begin to exercise after the baby is born?

As soon as her doctor will allow. She can begin almost immediately with isometric stomach-strengthening routines, which will help her to strengthen those weakened muscles without injuring herself. After a few weeks, with her doctor's permission, she should take up most of the routine exercises I recommend for people with common backache.

Which part of the whole child-bearing experience is hardest on the back?

Surprisingly, the worst time is usually after the baby is born. Not only because of the way the birth itself stretches various muscles and ligaments and saps some of the mother's strength, but also because of what a new mother goes through in caring for her baby – all that lifting of the child and its equipment, bending over the crib, doing the laundry, and so on. But all these hazards to her back can be greatly reduced if she prepares herself for them through exercise, good postural habits, and proper rest.

**From everything you've been saying, it sounds as though nobody
really needs to allow a bad back to interfere with his or her sex
life or prevent a couple from raising a family.**

That's exactly right. No question about it. Back pain does tend
to interrupt people's lives, sometimes with tragic consequences,
but there is usually no medical reason why this should happen.
If you understand what you're up against and know how to cope
with the pain – or, better still, learn how to prevent it from
happening – your back is no threat to your sex life and needn't
stop you from having a baby.

8. AS YOU GROW OLDER

If you are a middle-aged victim of common backache and feel trapped by the prospect of a lifetime of discomfort and misery, I have some encouraging words for you: as you grow older, your back will almost certainly get better, and if you live long enough, you'll outlive your back pain.

Most backache sufferers, of course, assume that their spines are in for the opposite experience – a lifetime of deterioration.

Happily, good old Mother Nature commonly treats us all better than that. Unless you find yourself among the small minority who suffer backache from one of the less common afflictions, you can take comfort from the statistics which show conclusively that most aching backs get better all by themselves when their owners are around seventy.

Unhappily, few physicians ever reveal this good news to their patients. Why is that? I suspect many doctors become so engrossed with the immediate situation that they never get around to discussing the patient's long-term prospects. Also, I think doctors are often wary of raising false expectations in the minds of patients who are likely to experience quite a number of painful episodes before their backs finally begin to give them less trouble.

As well, there are some afflictions associated with aging which affect a minority of the population but get so much public attention they contribute to the myth that backache is inevitable during old age. One notable example these days is osteoporosis, a widely discussed condition that is greatly feared – often needlessly. It's true that middle-aged women have special reason to be concerned about osteoporosis; it afflicts far more of them than it does middle-aged men. But it's also true that for most women and men, regardless of age, osteoporosis will never be a problem; only about 15 percent of the population suffer as a result of it, compared to the 80 percent who suffer from common backache at some time in their lives.

If I were to apportion space in this chapter to afflictions purely on the basis of the number of aging people who suffer from them, osteoporosis would rate far less space than I have given to it. But it's something that concerns many people and I believe they are entitled to be told everything they want to know about it. And so I deal fully with all the questions I am commonly asked about this condition. This discussion should reassure readers that osteoporosis is not an inevitable source of trouble or pain.

The amount of space allotted to other less common causes of backache is also out of proportion to the frequency of their occurrence, for the same reason.

I hope that, by the end of this chapter, you will have a better idea of how the aging process actually affects your back. And if only one message stays with you, let it be my opening statement: *Most people's back pain really does disappear as they grow older.*

You say backs get better with age, but I know lots of old people with stiff backs and joints, and stooped shoulders, and all sorts of aches and pains.

That's true. But most of their aches and pains come from other causes, mostly in other parts of their bodies. And don't overlook the fact that being stiff and feeling sore are not the same thing. The aging process that makes your back stiff also keeps your facet joints from moving as much, and so they cause you less pain.

Your back continues to undergo wear and tear, but you don't feel its effects nearly as much. So the stiffening of your back with age has a beneficial effect.

Also as you grow older, your whole pace of living slows down. As you place fewer demands on your body, your back gets extra rest and it's less likely to feel painful from normal use.

Of course there are exceptions to the rule. Just the other day, I met a woman of seventy-nine who had just experienced her very first attack of back pain. But she's in a real minority. It's much more common to see people who had back pain in their earlier years and got better as they grew older. This observation has been borne out repeatedly by studies all over the world.

I remember many occasions as a boy, when our family outings were cancelled at the last moment because of my father's back problems. He would simply have to take to his bed because his back was so painful. Years later, when I got into this business of telling people about back pain, I often said that backs get better with age, and of course I said so in my first book. When *The Back Doctor* came out, my father, who was then about eighty years old, called me up and said, "I don't think it's right for you to go around saying such a thing without consulting your father."

"Okay," I said, "what happened to your back pain?"

"Well," he said, "it got better."

Are you saying that someone can just ignore proper back care and still wind up eventually with a pain-free back?

In many cases, that's true. Mother Nature will always try to do her best for you, no matter how you neglect yourself. But to increase your chances of having a pain-free back in later years, and to avoid a lot of misery along the way, you should keep yourself in reasonable physical condition.

How would you define "reasonable physical condition"?

I'm talking mainly now about back and abdominal muscles. It's hardly surprising that a person reaching, say, age seventy finds it difficult to begin developing muscular strength.

People who have kept their muscles in good condition throughout their lives will find it much easier to improve their muscle tone in their older years, and that extra strength is important to protect their backs.

There are two reasons why it's difficult, late in life, to take up exercise for the first time. For one thing, you lack the habits that would help you get into an effective routine; for another, you lack the necessary muscle tissue. If you are going to exercise for the sake of your back, you need to pay special attention to your belly muscles and those ridges of muscle that run down each side of your spine – the paraspinal muscles.

Picture a seventy-year-old man with a pot belly and weak muscles around his mid-section. That extra weight out front is pulling on his spine, and he hasn't the muscles to protect his back from the strain. He's not just a candidate for back pain, he probably has some pain already.

And he could have avoided that problem by doing regular back exercises as a younger man?

To a great extent, yes, and it will be very difficult for him to start now.

What if he had started years ago and then stopped? Could he expect to start again with any success?

Certainly the more he exercised over the years the better his chances of resuming the habit. But it's one thing to keep in shape all your life and quite another thing to get back into shape once you've let yourself go. In our exercise clinic at the Canadian Back Institute we see a lot of middle-aged and older people who have delusions about their physical abilities. I call it the 65/25 Syndrome; it stands for body of 65, mind of 25. These people just don't understand, or refuse to believe, that their bodies, being older, will not respond as quickly as they once did to the resumption of exercise. Invariably they're shocked to discover they can't snap back into shape in six weeks of workouts. It takes a lot more work and a lot more time.

Is being in bad shape as much of a problem for women as it is for men?

It's a problem for both, but in overweight women, the extra pounds tend to be stored a little lower and a little further behind, which is less of a strain on the back. Of course, it's still important to be in good shape, and certainly a woman with back problems can benefit considerably from exercises that strengthen the abdomen and the paraspinal muscles.

I seem to be getting the message that there comes a time for some people when it would be pointless to exercise.

If an elderly person is able to exercise and has the desire, I wouldn't object. But others may find exercise a frustrating experience if they haven't done it before, and I would doubt their ability to keep it up. When you talk about exercise for people in their senior years, you've got to be practical and realistic.

What happens, then, to older people who have back trouble and can't or won't exercise?

Fortunately, nature is still on their side. Even without exercise, as I said earlier, the joints and discs will still stiffen up with age, making the back pain disappear. In the meantime, while the pain persists, there is a place for corsets or other forms of temporary support that will help you through a bad time. And we can all practice proper body mechanics – the right way to stand and sit, for example.

What about other causes of back pain besides wear and tear? Aren't there some to which older people are especially susceptible?

Yes, there are two that are particularly noteworthy. One is osteoporosis, which we can talk about in a moment. The other is acquired spinal stenosis, which we discussed earlier, designating it as Type Four back pain.

As you'll remember, acquired spinal stenosis is a condition where the size of the spinal canal is reduced by a chronically bulging disc, bony overgrowth, or a combination of the two. The narrowing of the passage itself doesn't necessarily cause trouble, but it may make it difficult for blood vessels to supply the nerves that control the muscles in your legs. The result is a condition called *cauda equina* claudication.

In a typical case, the backache isn't a major problem; it's the legs that are most painful. And even the legs are fine when resting. But after a few minutes' walk, they feel strange – cold, rubbery, or numb – and the person has to sit down and rest for several minutes. *Cauda equina* claudication affects the elderly more often than other age groups because their bodies have been in use long enough for bulging discs and bony growths to develop in the spinal canal.

An uncle of mine can't walk very far without his legs becoming very painful. His doctor told me the problem was a poor blood supply to the legs. Is that the problem you've just described?

No. But, because the symptoms are similar, it's often hard to tell whether the person with that complaint is suffering from poor blood supply to the nerves in the back, which is *cauda equina* claudication, or limited blood supply to the muscles of the legs themselves, which is vascular claudication.

In a physical examination, the two conditions can appear almost identical, and so we employ several tests to help with the diagnosis. Some of the tests done to confirm claudication brought on by spinal stenosis are in fact designed to rule out vascular insufficiency in the legs.

The key to the direct diagnosis of *cauda equina* claudication is the CT scan, which allows us to check the diameter of the spinal canal and detect the long-standing disc bulges or bony growths that can narrow the space. Before the CT scan was available, the only way we could get some idea of the size of the canal was to obtain a myelogram, which involves injecting radiopaque fluid into the nerve sac around the *cauda equina* and X-raying the critical area.

Apart from what we can learn through these diagnostic investigations, one of the clinical differences I have noted is that patients with trouble in the back may get the most relief when they rest in a specific position – often one that involves sitting bent forward or with one knee drawn up – whereas people with poor blood supply to the legs get relief by resting in any position.

Incidentally, the diagnosis can become particularly tricky when a patient with simple Type One or Type Two back pain also suffers from poor blood supply to his legs. The symptoms may sound like *cauda equina* claudication, when in fact the patient can have two entirely unrelated problems: simple back trouble, plus vascular claudication.

Obviously, the two types of claudication must be treated quite differently. *Cauda equina* claudication is treated surgically to enlarge the spinal canal and make more room for the nerves and their blood supply. However, as I mentioned earlier, we don't operate on a case of spinal stenosis just because the canal is narrow; we perform surgery only when that narrowing causes pressure on the nerves.

Treatment of the vascular type of claudication may require surgery directly on the blood vessels in the legs.

You also mentioned osteoporosis as an affliction that affects older people. What exactly is it?

It's a thinning of the bone, which commonly occurs with age. When you hear the term osteoporosis, don't think "disease"; it is just Doctor for a process that happens to virtually everyone who grows old. Most people are never aware it has happened to them, since only a minority of the population ever develops osteoporosis that's painful or disabling. The great majority of cases remain undiagnosed because the bone-thinning causes no problems. Technically, osteoporosis exists – quite harmlessly – in the spines of most middle-aged and older people.

Then I could have osteoporosis without feeling any pain?

That's right. The condition itself doesn't hurt. Pain occurs only when other problems develop, as we'll see later.

Does that thinning of bones take place only in the the spine?

No, it occurs in most other bones as well. For example, medical researchers have found that in people over eighty, the walls of a normal thigh bone are reduced in thickness by as much as 50 percent. The outside diameter of the bone remains the same but the thickness of the walls is reduced from the inside – just the opposite of what happens when a tree grows by adding an outside layer or "ring" of wood year after year.

If you're over forty, some of the bones in your body may already have walls that are thinner than they once were. They're thickest when you're in your late twenties or early thirties, and they begin to thin out some time after age forty. The space inside, previously occupied by bone, is filled up partly by marrow but mostly by fat. If you find this whole idea frightening, you should understand that it's just as normal for your bones to change over the years as it is for your skin to wrinkle or your hair to turn gray.

Osteoporosis is like a worn-out pair of jeans. They may get thin at the knees, but as long as they don't tear, they're still serviceable. Obviously, however, the thin material is more likely to give way under strain than when it was new, and just as you have to be careful with a worn pair of pants, you have to be careful with a back that has osteoporosis.

What causes osteoporosis?

We don't know the cause, but we do know it's related to aging and it affects some people much more than others. In many cases, it just seems to come on gradually as the person gets older. Other contributing factors are: a calcium deficiency; in women, an estrogen deficiency; smoking; heavy drinking; lack of exercise.

Specific diseases can upset the system and bring on osteoporosis. For example, your doctor might find you have hyper-thyroidism, a chronically overactive thyroid gland, which can decrease the calcium content of your bones and hasten the onset of osteoporosis. So, if a doctor finds you have osteoporosis, a complete medical examination is in order, so that any disease can be either ruled out or detected and treated.

When does osteoporosis become painful?

That will happen when the bone of a vertebra gets so thin that it cracks or crushes just from the weight it normally bears. The drum-shaped bodies of the vertebrae are made of porous bone, full of holes like a sponge. This spongy bone is not unique to the spine (your heels, for instance, are made of the same stuff) but it's quite different from, say, your shin bones or your ribs. Now, when osteoporosis sets in, the holes in those sponge-like bones grow larger. As you would expect, the more porous the bone becomes the weaker it gets. When it reaches the point where it's too weak to support the weight of the body, a vertebra can collapse.

You mean one of the bones will just suddenly give way?

That's right. The collapse can be triggered by something as innocuous as a sneeze or a cough.

A crushed vertebra sounds terribly painful.

You bet it is. It produces the kind of acute pain you get with any broken bone, and this pain usually lasts about six weeks, until healing is complete. That pain is often the first indication of a problem caused by osteoporosis.

Are there permanent effects, even after the crushed vertebra has healed?

Not usually. The healed fractures become pain free, and the function of the spine returns to normal. Sometimes the vertebral bodies are squeezed down unevenly, so that they are narrower at the front than at the back, and that part of the spine is tipped forward, creating the so-called "dowager's hump" you see in some elderly people – usually in women but sometimes in men as well.

Further collapse, or the involvement of several vertebrae, may also affect the alignment of the facet joints, which may therefore wear more rapidly and cause trouble. Also, if a disc happens to bulge against a vertebra weakened by osteoporosis, it may push right into the thin, spongy bone, and that, too, can be painful.

Is it true that women are more likely than men to be affected by osteoporosis?

Yes, they are. Most research indicates that, in proportion to body weight, a typical woman has about 30 percent less bone mass than a typical man. And so, if a man and a woman both experienced the natural thinning out of the bones at the same rate, the woman would suffer the consequences much sooner. Furthermore, women are more often afflicted by an accelerated type of osteoporosis.

For reasons we don't understand, this type afflicts Caucasian women more than those of other races. According to one recent continent-wide study, 25 percent of white women in North America over the age of sixty have one or more broken bones associated with osteoporosis.

Earlier you mentioned that smoking and heavy drinking contribute to osteoporosis. How does that happen?

We're not sure of the exact mechanism, but we think it has something to do with the body's hormonal regulating system, which controls the storage, distribution, and use of calcium. Normally, calcium is taken out of the gut, stored in the bone, and then released from there as needed for regulation of specific body functions, such as normal nerve conduction. As the blood passes through the kidneys, the calcium is routinely filtered out and some is recycled for repeated use.

This process may break down for several reasons. The kidneys may fail to recirculate the calcium. Or there may not be enough calcium getting into the system in the first place. Or, on the other hand, too much calcium may be released from the bones into the general circulation, causing an overload that is corrected through a greater than normal excretion of the mineral.

So the hormones that regulate the calcium level will fail if you drink heavily or smoke?

Not fail, exactly, but there is a strong chance they will become less effective. And this raises a point that I'm sure a lot of people don't know: the bones in your body are being renewed constantly. In fact, they are completely exchanged about every seven years. Two different kinds of cells are involved in this process. One cell, called the osteoblast, generates new bone, while another cell, the osteoclast, eats up the old bone and sends its various components off into the system. It's nature's way of replacing material that's worn down, worn out, or damaged. For instance, it's this process that enables facet joints to reshape themselves when the discs in your spine narrow, as I described earlier.

Of course there has to be a balance between the processes of tearing down and building up. If you have too much bone mass it will get in the way, and if you have too little it won't provide adequate support. Certain hormones must be present in proper quantities to regulate the cellular activity that removes, repairs, and replaces normal bone.

Throughout their early years, most people's bodies manage to maintain the proper balance between making and removing bone. But as they grow older, the process falters because of a hormonal imbalance (a common cause in women after the menopause) or for various other reasons, such as a deficiency of calcium or of additional bone-forming materials. As a result, the bone creation process slows down while the bone destruction keeps right on at its usual pace. And so the bones get thinner. That's osteoporosis.

What's the best treatment for osteoporosis?

Unfortunately, there is no fully effective treatment for osteoporosis, once it has developed. It can be arrested, and in a few patients it can be partially reversed but not fully corrected. The best strategy, then, is prevention. You can increase your chances of avoiding the problem by maintaining or increasing your calcium intake, exercising, drinking alcohol only moderately or not at all, and not smoking.

You said "maintaining or increasing your calcium intake" as though everybody were likely to develop a calcium deficiency.

The fact is that most people do have a calcium deficiency, at least in North America, where the problem has been studied extensively. To keep their bones in good shape, men and pre-menopausal women need at least 1000 mg of elemental calcium a day. Mothers who are breast-feeding and women who have gone through menopause need about 1500 mg a day. But according to most calculations, the usual intake in North America is only about 400 to 500 mg a day. In other words, most men and young women on this continent are getting only half the calcium they need and most older women are getting only a third of what they require.

Does that mean everybody ought to drink a lot more milk?

That would be one solution, but a lot of people can't or won't do it. To get enough extra calcium from milk, most adults would have to drink about two more eight-ounce glasses than they now consume; post-menopausal women and breast-feeding mothers would need about three to four glasses a day beyond what they already take as part of their regular diet. That could be especially difficult for older people, whose systems don't tolerate milk readily.

What foods besides milk contain calcium?

There is calcium in other dairy products, such as cheese and yogurt. It's also contained in leafy green vegetables, kidney beans, and canned salmon and sardines, especially in the soft bones. It is possible to get a sufficient quantity of calcium from your diet, but not many people eat enough of the proper foods regularly to get the calcium they need.

What about calcium pills?

They can help prevent osteoporosis from developing. Men and pre-menopausal women should take about 500 mg of calcium a day, to supplement the calcium they get in their normal diet. Older women and breast-feeding mothers should take twice that amount.

Is there a danger of overdosing on calcium pills?

Under normal conditions, it's not possible to harm yourself by taking too much calcium by mouth, thanks to that natural control mechanism I described. The extra mineral just passes through the system and is discarded.

Can calcium pills help people who already have osteoporosis?

Yes, but since the process is not reversible simply with calcium treatment, the pills are useful only to stop it from getting worse.

Can extra hormones be prescribed to overcome the hormonal deficiency that leads to osteoporosis?

Estrogens, which are female hormones, have been used quite

successfully to prevent the loss of bone in post-menopausal women. But there can be undesirable side effects – and estrogens don't reverse osteoporosis, either; the most they do is arrest it.

What sort of side effects does estrogen cause?

Taken by itself, estrogen increases the risk of cancer in the uterus. This risk can be eliminated if a woman is willing to take progesterone along with the estrogen. They are the two hormones in birth control pills, and when they are taken in cyclical doses they will re-establish menstruation. When menstruation returns, I recommend regular check-ups by a gynecologist.

Would that mean there is a chance of becoming pregnant?

No, there's no chance of that. But there are other considerations. You can't prevent osteoporosis simply by adding some estrogen for a month or two. It has to be a long-term commitment. If you start taking estrogen-progesterone replacement and then stop it, your bone loss will rapidly return to its normal rate, and you will be no further ahead. If you took estrogen for, say, two years after menopause and then stopped, your chance of developing osteoporosis would be the same from then on, as if you never took the hormone replacement at all.

And yet we hear a lot these days about the benefits of estrogen.

Yes, and that worries me. Drug companies have always tried to sell estrogen by persuading doctors to prescribe it for their patients. But many doctors resisted the idea, for the reasons I just mentioned. More recently, advertisements lauding estrogen have been aimed directly at the public, and many patients are asking their doctors to prescribe estrogen to help in the management of their osteoporosis.

Then what do you say to a patient who asks about estrogen?

I explain the pros and cons and I point out that it involves a decision that's not to be taken hastily or lightly.

Can't anything be done to treat people who have osteoporosis?

Curative treatment is still a doubtful proposition, but doctors have had some success with sodium fluoride, usually augmented by extra calcium and vitamin D. Incidentally, the amount of sodium fluoride prescribed is much greater than the amount added to drinking water to toughen children's teeth. The extra fluoride, combined with the calcium and vitamin D, can actually promote the formation of bone. However, some people respond to this treatment while others don't.

Fluoride should be administered only by a specialist who knows exactly what he's doing. In large doses it can cause nausea and gastro-intestinal bleeding, and it makes the bones brittle, leaving the patient susceptible to fractures in the hips and long bones. It may also produce the excessive formation of bone spurs.

On the positive side, fluoride is capable of toughening up the porous bone in the spine, preventing the rapid bone loss that might lead to the collapse of a vertebra.

Two other substances that have shown some promise are gland extracts called calcitonin and parathormone. But these hormones must be given by frequent injections, and the cost is substantial – with no assurance that the treatment will work and no convincing evidence that they can bring about a meaningful reduction in the number of fractures that occur.

I feel the research in this area is very promising. But at this point, there is no simple answer to the problem of treating osteoporosis.

You implied earlier that exercise might help. How does it relate to osteoporosis?

We don't know the whole answer, but it's been recognized for almost a century that your bones respond to use by getting stronger, in much the same way as your muscles do. And there is much more recent medical evidence that even light exercise, if it's done fairly regularly, can retard the loss of calcium.

Or, to be more exact, I should say studies show that people who exercise regularly seem to lose less calcium than those who don't exercise. Although I'm in favor of exercise, and the recent studies are certainly promising, I have to admit that it's hard to isolate the benefit of exercise from the effects of a generally healthy lifestyle. Many people who exercise regularly are also likely to avoid unhealthy habits, such as drinking heavily or smoking. And so, to be scientific about it, you have to ask: are people better off because they exercise or because they have developed healthy habits?

Incidentally, investigations into exercise have concentrated mainly on women, because of their special need to prevent calcium loss after menopause.

Then osteoporosis is less of a threat to women who are athletic?

That's not necessarily true. There is evidence that extremely strenuous workouts can upset the hormonal balance. Doctors have found that female athletes who run much more than twenty miles (32 km) per week may develop the condition known as amenorrhea. That is, they stop menstruating. The theory is that if the amount of body fat drops below a certain critical level, the body's production of estrogen also drops. In any case, the development of amenorrhea is a pretty clear indication that the hormonal levels are askew. And without the right balance, there's a greater risk of rapid osteoporosis. Researchers have found that a woman of twenty-five who exercises excessively – and here we're talking about someone training at an Olympic level – can suffer as much bone loss as an average woman would expect at age fifty.

Then the moral of this whole exercise story is moderation?

That's exactly right. Don't become sedentary, but don't become an exercise freak, either.

The most important point to make about osteoporosis is that a certain amount of bone loss is normal with aging. You can't prevent it entirely, but you don't need to, because it's unlikely to cause a problem. Excessive bone loss, on the other hand, is preventable, and if you let it develop to the point where it allows fractures causing pain or disability, you could be in for a lot of trouble.

What about other painful back conditions that develop as a person grows older?

One is degenerative scoliosis, another type of the spinal curvature we discussed earlier. It's different from the scoliosis that occurs in children, where the curvature is the result of an abnormal spinal growth.

Do we know what causes degenerative scoliosis?

Typically it results from an uneven pattern of wear and drying out in the disc. One side of the disc flattens down more than the other, so that it becomes wedge-shaped. Consequently, the spine tilts over toward the flatter side, causing a curvature.

Is degenerative scoliosis painful? How is it treated?

This form of scoliosis often puts increased pressure on the joints, discs, or nerves, causing pain that's virtually the same as common backache. The treatment is also the same: exercise, posture training, muscle strengthening, and in some instances surgery, if the narrowing between the vertebrae is so severe that the symptoms can't be relieved in any other way.

Are there other back conditions associated with aging that people should know about?

Another condition that's uncommon but worth noting is degenerative spondylolisthesis – an ailment that is easier to understand than it is to pronounce. "Spondyl" means "relating to the bones of the spine," and "listhesis" is a slip. For reasons no one understands, this problem occurs most often at a specific level of the lumbar spine in women over the age of forty-five. The facet joints connecting the fourth and fifth lumbar vertebrae are L-shaped and positioned to lock into place. (Anatomically there are five lumbar vertebrae, numbered downward, making Lumbar 5, or L_5 as it is usually called, the last movable segment before the pelvis.) In some people, as the joints wear with age, they flatten out, and the locking effect is lost. This means the entire fourth lumbar vertebra, now held only by the L_4-L_5 disc, is free to slide forward very slowly. When that happens, you get pain.

Can anything be done about this slippage?

Treatment is not always necessary. Sometimes with further aging the area stiffens up by itself, and when the movement stops, so does the pain. If the symptoms persist, they can sometimes be controlled by exercises that strengthen the belly muscles, so that they can take some of the load off the spine. However, when there is significant slippage because the joints have completely lost their ability to lock together, surgery may be the only way to go.

Is surgery likely to succeed in a case like that?

As a rule it will. Since the problem is clearly identified and the mechanical failure is quite local, a spinal fusion is usually a success-ful way of stopping the slippage. In this operation we span the distance between the two vertebrae with strips of bone, and in that way we fuse the fourth and fifth lumbar vertebrae into a single, longer bone. The joints above and below the fused area remain functional, with their lock mechanisms still working nor-mally. Of course movement at the L_4-L_5 space is gone, but that's the idea; otherwise the facet joints would remain unstable.

What about cancer of the spine as a source of back pain in older people?

Cancer can originate in the back in one of two locations. It can begin in the vertebral bone, or it can develop in the blood-forming tissue within the bone, that is the bone marrow. Either way, it's rare for cancer to originate in the spine; the occurrence rate is much less than for cancer of the lung, breast, or prostate.

What about cancer that spreads to the spine from somewhere else?

It is more common – or, I should say, less rare – to find the spine

affected by a cancer that has spread from some other part of
the body. But almost always, this cancer is diagnosed before it
reaches the back. And, for that reason, neither the patient nor
the doctor is inclined to regard the illness as a spinal problem,
but rather as a cancer that is becoming a threat throughout the
body.

In very rare instances, patients may complain of back pain that
turns out to be caused by cancer in the spine that spread there
from somewhere else even though the original source cannot be
identified. To give you some idea of how rare this is: out of the
more than 40,000 back patients I have examined, I've encountered
only three cases of this kind.

In short, if you don't have cancer anywhere else in your body,
your chances of having it in your spine are extremely remote,
whatever your age.

What kinds of cancer are likely to spread to the back?

Breast cancer is one. Another is cancer of the prostate, which,
as you know, is a problem for men in their older years. A third
is multiple myeloma, a cancer that may originate in the spine
but actually attacks the blood-forming cells of the bone marrow
in many parts of the body. The incidence of these last two cancers
increases as people grow older. Again, I must stress that, although
the numbers go up with age, the possibility of spinal cancer is
still very unlikely.

**As unlikely as it may be, if I did have cancer in my back, what
would the symptoms be?**

Nobody should jump to that conclusion, but I will mention two
symptoms. First, a pain that is constant, even at rest. By that I
mean a pain that remains unchanged no matter what you do
to seek relief. Bending backward, stooping forward, sitting, lying
down – nothing makes any difference to the pain. Second, a pain
that has been present for a relatively short time. Malignancies
of this sort progress rapidly, and if you have had the same problem
in your back for, say, one or two years, it is not cancer. It is probably
just one of the common types of back pain. But if your back is

bothering you and you don't know what's wrong, see your doctor. Chances are you'll gain peace of mind, as well as receiving advice about the appropriate remedy for whatever the problem may be.

If you suspected a patient's back pain was caused by cancer, how would you proceed?

I would order several diagnostic procedures. I'd want a series of blood tests conducted to look for the chemical changes that occur when bone is being destroyed by a malignant tumor. I would also order certain X-ray studies, such as a CT scan or perhaps a different type of bone scan in which a radioactive material is injected into the system. This material becomes incorporated briefly into the structure of the bone. On the scan, the doctor can see an increased amount of the material in any area where there is excessive bone reaction. That doesn't necessarily mean there's a tumor there, but it does indicate that the body is reacting – to something. And this can be a valuable clue in the search for what is wrong.

What advice do you have for people who are worried that cancer may be the cause of their back pain?

The first thing I want them to understand is that cancer as a cause of back pain is extremely rare. But if they have any apprehension, they should see a doctor. He may use the tests I just described, although I must point out that I don't use them routinely in my own practice, because they simply aren't necessary. I emphasize that point because I would hate to think this discussion might give anyone the idea that their doctor wasn't being thorough enough if he ruled out cancer without conducting the tests.

How would you summarize what older people should know about back problems?

We've spent quite a bit of time talking about the back pain some older people experience from causes other than wear and tear. It is important to remember that these afflictions are very uncommon. They make up only a small fraction of all backache cases. And we have effective remedies for most of them. One exception is osteoporosis. As a natural process that can become excessive, it exemplifies the adage about an ounce of prevention being worth a pound of cure.

The most important point of all, however, is one I made right at the beginning of this discussion: for nearly everybody, mechanical back pain gets better with age.

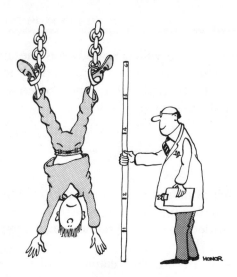

9. AEROBICS, HEEL-HANGING, AND OTHER AMUSEMENTS

Among the steady stream of people who come to me with back problems, there are always some who are looking for shortcuts to recovery.

They want my opinion, if not my approval, of devices such as gravity traction outfits or weight-lifting machines, and various "in" exercises such as yoga, as means of treating their pain or improving their backs. I'm sure some of them feel I'm being deliberately evasive when I decline either to endorse one of these alternatives without qualification or to condemn it as worthless.

My position usually lies somewhere between the two extremes. There is no such thing as *the* treatment that helps everyone. The remedy that provides dramatic relief to Patient A may prove utterly ineffective for Patient B. Knowing that, I am pragmatic enough to say, "If it doesn't hurt and it's not harmful, try it." On that basis, and if it helps the patient feel better, I'm delighted.

And of course backs do get better by themselves. Acute attacks inevitably subside, and even chronic pain recedes, in time, as a person ages and the body adjusts. And so with any treatment that is followed by apparent improvement or recovery, you have to ask: "What made the patient's back get better? Was it the therapy, or was the pain about to disappear anyway?"

Those are questions to which nobody has the answers. But I do have answers to the questions my patients most often ask about faddish exercises and therapies sometimes touted as the ultimate solutions to the painful back.

What do you think of those new devices that are supposed to relieve backache by letting you hang upside down, by your heels or in a sitting position, for several minutes each day?

They are forms of an age-old treatment called gravity traction, and the only things new about them are the upside-down position, the big price tag, and the questionable claims of success. As a concept, gravity traction is at least as old as medieval times, when a patient would be fastened, right side up, to a ladder, with weights attached to his feet, to pull down on his spine and thus relieve his back pain.

The idea of gravity traction is to provide more pull on the back than can be generated by conventional traction. In the conventional method, a patient lies on his back, wearing a waist-belt attached to weights that hang over the end of the bed and pull steadily on the spine. To keep the weights from pulling the person onto the floor, the foot of the bed is usually tipped up slightly. Even so, there's a limit to the amount of pull that can be exerted without dragging the patient off the bed, and a lot of the benefit of that pull is wasted by the friction of the apparatus and the patient against the sheets.

Does bed traction actually relieve back pain?

Sometimes it does, but probably only because it keeps the patient in bed and resting. If you put anybody with back pain in a comfortable position for a week, chances are the person will get better. I suspect the traction has very little to do with the patient's recovery. But a few doctors who believe in the value of traction decided they could overcome the friction problem and at the same time increase the traction by using the weight of the person's own body to provide the pull, suspending him in mid-air wearing a chest harness somewhat like a parachutist's gear. To give the body a chance to adjust gradually to the gravitational pull without pain or harm, the patient starts out flat on a tilting bed. Then, with each successive treatment, the slope of the bed is increased until the patient is virtually upright.

Incidentally, I tried that type of traction for my own back problem, but it didn't work out very well. For some reason, no matter how tightly I was strapped in, my body kept slipping through the harness, and I soon abandoned the whole idea.

Maybe the same harness problems gave somebody the idea of hanging by the heels instead.

Could be. That variation apparently got started in California in the 1970s. But it never really caught on until 1980, with the release of a movie called *American Gigolo*, in which the star, Richard Gere, practiced gravity traction, using boots fixed to an overhead bar. Soon, people all over the continent were suspending themselves upside down.

What happens, exactly, when gravity traction is applied – upside down or otherwise?

One of the problems is that nobody really knows. When it's used regularly, gravity traction does relieve back pain for some people. But we're not sure why. Maybe it relieves spasm in the muscles by stretching them and inducing them to relax. Or perhaps it counteracts pressure on the small joints of the spine. It's possible that if you pull with enough force on the low back, the facet joints that are sore from being jammed together will separate slightly, easing the pressure and reducing the pain. The action is the same as the one I mentioned during our discussion of neck problems. It's also possible that a strong pull on the outer fibers of a bulging lumbar disc will be enough to reduce the size of the bulge and decrease the local irritation. All these things could happen, at least while the traction is being applied.

But the evidence in favor of gravity traction isn't conclusive?

No, the possibilities I just mentioned are speculative. The problem is the size and strength of the spine in the lower back. Several studies have been done with special X-ray investigations to measure the difference, if any, in the shape of a disc's shell before and after gravity traction. According to some reports, the treatment seemed to have reduced the bulging; other reports say it had no apparent effect. Certainly the reaction is not uniform, and the weight of evidence suggests that gravity traction doesn't produce any permanent change. The most you can say for it is that it seems to help some people's backs sometimes.

But weren't the newer forms of gravity traction developed by reputable medical experts?

Many were, but that doesn't automatically make them right. Furthermore, if you find it helpful to stretch your body with gravity traction, you're not necessarily better off upside down than right side up. I've read claims that the inverted position is beneficial to the heart, lungs, and brain, but I have also seen studies indicating that hanging with your head down can produce serious side effects, such as aggravating glaucoma from the extra pressure on the eyeballs, or contributing to high blood pressure. In my view, gravity traction owes its popularity more to slick marketing than to proven statistics. The result is that people are willing to pay sometimes as much as $1,000 for an apparatus that lets them hang upside down exactly as they could, free of charge, from a jungle gym in a children's playground.

Aren't you being a little harsh, considering that some people would want to use the equipment in private, at home, and have apparently found merit in this form of treatment?

My concern here is not the potential benefits but the aggressive manner in which gravity traction is merchandized. If you read the promotional literature carefully you will see just how much hype it contains. You'll find it filled with extravagant statements that are impossible to pin down: "Many orthopedic surgeons are prescribing it"; "Nine out of ten sufferers report immediate results ... dramatic relief during their first two-minute session"; a "breakthrough [that] applies space-age technology"; "state-of-the-art"; and so on.

To me, those sound like pitches from a snake-oil salesman, up-dated for the 1980s.

Are you saying the manufacturers are making questionable claims?

Let's say they do a pretty thorough job of mixing fact with fancy while overlooking recognized medical knowledge. Here's an example from one pamphlet:

Q. What about stress-related factors?
A. Chronic pain is often associated with debilitating emotional stress, muscle tension and physical fatigue – triggering states of fear, anxiety and depression, rage, frustration. . . .

What they say up to that point is perfectly true, as we have already discussed in this book. But then the brochure goes on:

Relaxing muscle spasm and releasing disc compression inter-rupts the pain cycle – while defusing stress and tension.

First, assuming for the moment that gravity traction actually does "release" your disc compression (whatever that means) there is no proof that this will interrupt the pain cycle and that stress and tension will be "defused" (which I assume is Hype for "relieved").

Second, even if these results are achieved, you have to wonder: will the traction provide more than a few minutes' relief?

And third, interrupting your pain cycle doesn't come anywhere near *altering* it. As long as it's still there, it will soon be back in full force, causing the same old agony and spasm. Yet nothing in the literature concedes that the relief is likely to be temporary.

Another statement in a brochure suggests that gravity traction can be used to treat an acute sports injury. It is saying, in effect, that if you tear a ligament in your neck, give it a good pull with gravity traction and it will get better. That's not true. Treating an acute ligament injury with traction will be painful, and it makes no more sense than pulling on a newly sprained ankle or pounding a bruise with a hammer.

The silliest claim of all is presented in some good old rough-and-tumble comparative advertising in the Coke-and-Pepsi tradi-tion. A drawing shows two young men hanging head down. One is hanging by his heels, from a competitor's product consisting of a horizontal bar and heavy ankle straps. The other young man, using the advertiser's product, is hanging from his waist, with his thighs across the seat of what looks like an expensive version of a backyard swing. The copy reads in part:

> Medical specialists agree that the key to alleviating low-back pain is to *flatten* the lumbar curve and *stretch* the spine... [emphasis theirs]

That is startling news to *this* medical specialist, who regards a moderate lumbar curve as healthy and natural. But there's more:

> Computerized results prove that [our product] flattens the lumbar curve and stretches the spine an average of *2.7 inches more* than [the rival product] [emphasis theirs].

Never mind whether that claim is actually true, and let's not bother asking why a computer was needed to make such simple measurements. Let's consider the long-term implications for the gravity-traction industry. Will future, improved models of these devices stretch people's spines even more – an additional four, six, eight, twelve inches? Are we on the threshold of creating a whole new race of people who are totally free of back pain and stand eight feet tall? You have to wonder: where were these promoters when the Spanish Inquisition needed them?

But, all joking aside, it must be confusing for back pain sufferers who face that kind of sales pitch.

Confusing, yes, and if it diverts them from more effective long-term management of their backs, it's doing them a disservice. I'm not opposed to gravity traction in all cases, but it does have its limitations, and people should be aware of them. We do know that in nearly four cases out of five, neck traction – manual or mechanical – is effective in relieving acute muscle spasm. And it is possible that gravity traction does the same thing for the low back in spite of the greater rigidity there.

But, as I have said, it doesn't help everybody. And certainly it is not the panacea it's sometimes made out to be. Common sense will tell you that no single form of treatment is capable of relieving every kind of neck or low-back problem, regardless of its nature or cause, or what stage it has reached.

If your problem is common backache, hanging upside down isn't going to harm your spine, although it may not be good for other parts of your body. But when it is suggested to me that there are long-term benefits to be gained from a few minutes of gravity traction each day, that's when they lose me.

It seems to me that the greatest long-term benefit from gravity traction may accrue not to the people who are using the devices but to the companies that are selling them.

Would you make the same criticism of the more conventional machines people are using for exercise and body-building – cycling machines, rowing machines, weight-lifting machines, and so on?

No, I wouldn't, although I do have some reservations about them. Assuming you apply sensible training methods, warming up for each workout and practicing moderation, I see nothing wrong with using exercise machines. However, if you intend to exercise without the supervision of a competent trainer, I suggest you read up on the particular machine you intend to use, or discuss it with a qualified physical therapist or fitness specialist, so that you understand the correct procedures and safeguards.

The main hazard is that whether an exercise routine is beneficial or detrimental, an exercise machine will magnify the effect. If you do everything right, the machine will magnify the benefits you get from it; but if you do things wrong, it will magnify your pain.

I'll give you an example. Most popular exercise machines use variable weights to provide tension and resistance for muscle development. One standard routine on these machines is an exercise intended to strengthen the muscles in the backs of your thighs. You lie on your stomach with your legs straight and your calves under a padded bar. Then you bend your knees. If you do it right, this routine strengthens your hamstring muscles. But if you overload the weight on the bar, you force yourself to work too hard at bending your knees. Instinctively, you will arch your back to gain extra leverage. That extra strain on your back is likely to cause pain if your facet joints are worn and hurt every time they are squeezed together.

To avoid the unwanted effects in this case you start with a lighter load. It will take you a little longer to get the results you want, but you will avoid a great deal of unnecessary discomfort. If you are considering exercising with any sort of machine, remember: while it's bad enough to do any exercise improperly, it's worse to do one whose ill effects will be magnified.

What about aerobic exercise for people with back problems?

I see nothing basically wrong with strenuous aerobic exercise if you're already in good shape. But most of us aren't. Aerobic routines require little strength but a lot of flexibility and stamina. They won't do much to prevent or overcome common backache. In fact, the impact of jumping up and down for twenty minutes may be enough to make your back sore. And the forceful bending and twisting movements that are part of so many programs will add to your discomfort. Aerobic exercises are designed to condition your heart and lungs, but they may not suit your needs as a back-pain sufferer. There are "low impact" routines available that provide good stimulation for the heart and lungs without placing unnecessary strain on your spine.

If you get into any heavy exercises without considering their effect on your spine, you're asking for trouble. If aerobic exercises are what you want, choose some that will also help strengthen or at least protect your back – swimming or riding an exercise bike, for example.

Then you approve of aquatic exercise?

Yes, water is a good medium for exercise – you can put your muscles through their paces without the effect of gravity, keeping the load off your spine while gaining all the benefits of stretching, strengthening, and aerobic routines. Almost any kind of swimming is helpful to back patients, although the particular approach best for you will depend on the exact nature of your problem. A well-done pool program is an excellent form of therapy – a good way to augment the more specific back exercises I'll be detailing in my final chapter.

I have only two reservations when my patients tell me they have started swimming to help their backs. For one thing, I wonder if they realize that swimming will help them only if they follow a schedule of exercises. Just getting into the water to float around is not enough. Also, I wonder if they will stick with the routine. Some patients who start pool therapy in a rehabilitation department often do well until they are discharged, and then they drop their exercise program because they don't have ready access to another swimming pool. All they're doing, of course, is shirking the responsibility for their own rehabilitation. Most communities these days have pools open to the public and, in any case, you can exercise without water, or, for that matter, without equipment of any kind. You certainly don't need a swimming pool of your own to keep your back in shape.

I recall you didn't recommend jogging as an exercise for people with back problems.

Jogging provides no direct benefit to your vertebral column or to the back and stomach muscles that are important in maintaining a healthy spine. One study even suggests that joggers should have strong stomach muscles before they start running, to reduce the risk of backache. In other words, if you go jogging, you should have reasons other than wanting to control your back pain.

What do you think of yoga as a means of avoiding or overcoming back trouble?

I consider yoga interesting and useful. It is certainly not a fad. As therapy for back problems I find it a healthy combination of exercise and mental discipline. It's no panacea, but then no form of treatment is.

Yoga exercises don't do much to increase a person's strength, although they often help flexibility. On the other hand, yoga's relaxation and meditation techniques, involving deep breathing and other routines, are excellent pain-control mechanisms. In that way, they resemble some of the therapy provided by pain clinics to relieve muscle tension and diminish a patient's focus on pain.

There are, however, certain things about yoga that require caution if you are a backache victim. In performing yoga exercises, you will be putting your body, including your back, through a wide range of movements – stretching muscles in your groin and thighs as well as along your spine. These routines are good unless they overload an inflamed facet joint in the low back or put too much pressure or torque on a worn disc. Then the exercise will aggravate your back pain. For instance, the cobra, an extension maneuver, is not a wise choice for someone with Type One trouble. The shoulder stand can be a real killer if you have Type Two difficulties. Whatever your problem may be, I assume you will make the obvious distinction between a recurrence of your typical pain and the discomfort and normal aches you feel the day after any new physical routine. If an exercise causes a flare-up, strike it off your list, at least temporarily, and try it again, carefully, some time when your back is feeling better.

You should understand, too, that yoga is not designed to provide specific help for your back. Therefore, if you came to me and said, "I want something to help my back," I wouldn't likely say, "Well, go and do yoga." On the other hand, if you came and said, "I want to try yoga – do you think it's all right?" I would approve, unless I knew a particular reason why you shouldn't participate.

But, as with any new routine, the more you find out about it, the better you will be able to judge whether it has potential benefits and, if so, decide if it should become part of your individual program of back care.

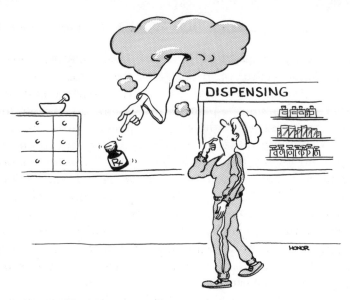

10. "MAGIC POTIONS" OR ALTERNATIVE TREATMENTS

In my practice, I keep encountering a few otherwise intelligent people who are convinced that, some day soon, someone will produce an instant cure for common backache. And I never cease to be amazed at those who believe a magic potion has already been discovered but is being suppressed by the medical establishment.

One phone call I received from a doctor in Florida was particularly disheartening. Would I mind telling him the name of the "miracle drug" I was using up in Canada? He said a former patient of mine, now living in Florida, had come asking for the same injection that I had administered to him about a year earlier. The doctor hadn't heard of any drug available in the U.S. that could cause a patient's backache to disappear instantly, leaving him pain free for an entire year. Now that the pain had returned, both doctor and patient were anxious, naturally, for a second magic dose.

When I heard the man's name, I realized part of the story was true. This patient had come to see me two or three times, complaining of low-back pain radiating to the top of his right buttock. My examination showed that the primary cause was simple

Type One facet joint pain with much of the discomfort referred to a trigger point on the bony ridge above the sacroiliac joint.

Originally, I prescribed routine exercises to strengthen his abdominal muscles, but the pain persisted, and so I decided that a little temporary relief might alter the pattern and encourage the man to continue working towards lasting recovery. Offering the patient no greater expectation than that, I injected a local short-acting anesthetic into the trigger point – a treatment, incidentally, that has been used by family doctors for decades.

The injection worked – dramatically. So well, in fact, that I never saw the man again. Soon after his last visit, he left Canada and settled in Florida, where, as I now was learning, he had evidently spent a year free of pain.

As I recounted the history to my colleague, I could almost hear the disappointment rising at the other end of that long-distance line.

"Sorry," I had to say, "but I have no magic potion for backache." The man had simply been the beneficiary of a lucky coincidence in which the temporary relief of my injection happened to combine with the spontaneous improvement of his back pain. The best I could suggest was that the doctor repeat the treatment and see what happened. Another shot of local anesthetic couldn't possibly do the patient any harm, and, considering what the first injection had done, it might just help again.

I never did hear how it came out, but for all I know, there is a transplanted Canadian living in Florida today who still thinks he was treated with a miracle drug available only in his native land.

That wouldn't surprise me in the least. What does surprise me is that a colleague was willing to believe I'd found a miraculous treatment and had been quietly dispensing it to my patients here in Canada, without sharing my marvelous discovery with the rest of the medical community.

While I don't disparage any treatment that helps people's backs get better without undesirable side effects, I keep stressing the futility of their searching for that non-existent magic cure. The search is certain to lead to disappointment and – worse still – may distract them from the exercises and proper living habits that offer the best long-term solution to their problem.

Many drugs, devices, and therapeutic procedures currently

touted as cures for backache would receive little further attention or acclaim if more doctors provided their patients with a thorough understanding of back pain, helping them realize that the most effective treatment usually includes their own active participation in a continuing program of management.

Physiologically, many of these alternatives have little to recommend them. But they offer new hope to the patient who emerges from the doctor's office, having received a cursory examination, a hastily scribbled prescription, and the terse instruction: "Take some of these pills and see if you feel better."

Compared to that approach, almost any other sort of treatment must seem more promising, especially if it is sold with great enthusiasm and conviction by someone claiming to have helped thousands of others with the same problem.

Unfortunately, even doctors who try to be responsive to their patients' needs will sometimes leave a mistaken impression. I've learned that from listening to the patients who come to me after seeing someone else.

"I saw my own doctor," they'll say, "but he didn't do anything."

"What do you mean? Didn't he examine you?"

"Well, yes."

"And didn't he tell you what was wrong with your back?"

"Yes, but then he didn't do anything. He just said we'd have to wait and see."

What we have here is not an uncaring doctor but a simple failure to communicate. From my own professional experience I know that "wait and see" is often exactly the right thing to do. Acute attacks subside and backs do get better by themselves. But I also know how important it is for the doctor to make it clear that waiting is not the same as doing nothing. Any time it's necessary for me to tell a patient "wait and see," I take care to avoid giving the impression that I'm not interested in the patient's problem or that I can't think of what to do next.

When I do counsel a patient to just wait, I seldom object if he or she wants to try some alternative form of treatment during that time, provided that it's not dangerous and the person has a clear and realistic idea of its purpose, its potential, and its limitations.

In this chapter I discuss a variety of alternative therapies ranging from the useful to the useless. There are many more I don't mention, but I have tried to give some idea of the kinds that offer genuine relief and those that create only false hope. The term "magic potions" refers less to the offerings of the practitioners than to the unrealistic expectations in the mind of the anxious patient.

I've been told that an injection of chymopapain can cure backache and eliminate the need for back surgery. Could that be the miracle cure we've all been waiting for?

Not quite. Unlike injections used for temporary relief from pain or inflammation, chymopapain can be a permanent remedy but it is useful only for Type Three back pain, when the nerve is pinched by a bulging disc. It is a chemical derived from the papaya fruit, similar to the tenderizer you might use on a tough steak. The material is injected into the disc to soften the nucleus and relieve pressure on the nerve.

Many people have the mistaken idea that chymopapain dissolves the center, or nucleus, of the disc. Actually, it denatures the protein of the nucleus, transforming a hard bulge into a soft bulge by destroying the tissue's ability to retain water. Figuratively speaking, it's like turning a walnut into a marshmallow. Usually this transformation cannot even be detected on a CT scan because the shape of the lump remains the same; only its texture is changed.

The fact that chymopapain doesn't actually remove the lump is probably one reason why it won't relieve Type Two pain, which comes from the disc itself. The bulging disc still bulges, and it continues to create a problem by stretching the outer shell. In fact, by drying out the nucleus, the injection may actually accelerate the natural aging process of the disc, and over time produce Type One or Type Two pain.

Is chymopapain safe? I heard it was banned in the United States for several years.

In the hands of a competent and experienced doctor, chymopapain is at least as safe as surgery. It was taken off the market in the

United States as a result of a large scientific study that seemed to show that it had no beneficial effect. The drug was never actually banned. It was voluntarily withdrawn by the manufacturer until further tests could be carried out. Many doctors, continuing to believe the injection was useful, pressed for its reinstatement. Meanwhile, chymopapain remained available in Canada, and thousands of Americans crossed the border to receive the drug. Eventually, further investigation reconfirmed its benefits, and chymopapain was reintroduced into the U.S.

One good thing to come out of the careful evaluation was a better understanding of how chymopapain should be used. Many of the unsatisfactory results, and almost all the complications, come from an ill-advised selection of patients (that is, people whose back problems cannot be corrected by this treatment) and from poor injection techniques.

Then is chymopapain really an alternative to surgery in certain cases?

I don't consider chymopapain an alternative to surgery; I tell my patients it's a first step that may make subsequent treatment, including surgery, unnecessary. If you have Type Three pain, and I inject chymopapain, I do so with every hope that it will clear up your problem, so that you won't need an operation. Although its success rate overall is about 70 percent, chymopapain works well in some cases and not at all in others, for reasons we don't fully understand. If the injection fails to reduce the nerve-root irritation, the only thing to do is to move on to the second step, which is surgery. Whenever I recommend chymopapain I always make it clear that the treatment doesn't always work. And so we are talking about surgery if necessary, but not necessarily surgery.

There is another way to look at the issue. Because the indications for chymopapain injection and surgery are exactly the same, if you have a condition where one of those two treatments can't help you, the other can't either. It makes no sense to consider the injection if you have already been told that surgery will not help in your case. Chymopapain isn't non-specific therapy for back pain; it is a chemical method which can provide relief of symptoms from direct nerve-root pressure.

I imagine most people would rather have chymopapain than surgery.

That's true, but chymopapain can be a painful treatment, and it has its own complications, limitations, and uncertainties. Perhaps I can illustrate what I mean if I tell you about the experience of a woman I'll call Stacey Wilson. Five years before her second episode, I had seen Mrs. Wilson for an acute attack of back pain with definite signs of pressure on a nerve root supplying part of the right leg. She recovered slowly without surgery.

The second time, her back problem was accompanied by pain running into the left leg and the loss of function in a nerve root coming from the left side of the spine. The CT scan showed two bulging discs, one pressing a nerve to the right, the cause of her previous trouble, and one pressing a nerve to the left, the source of the new pain.

I decided to use chymopapain on both discs to relieve the acute pressure to the left from the one below and reduce the chance of future trouble to the right from the disc above. Surgery at both levels was possible but would have produced more trauma to the spine and resulted in more scarring.

I gave Mrs. Wilson the injections, in both of those troublesome discs, and for three days she enjoyed complete relief. At 4:45 A.M. on the fourth day, her back and left leg pain returned with a vengeance. She endured it for almost three hours, then called me at 7:30 in the morning. I had her readmitted to the hospital. I was not alarmed by the return of her pain, since chymopapain can be initially painful and, in some cases, it will continue to produce severe back spasms for weeks. But one aspect of her problem was worrisome: Mrs. Wilson's leg pain had also returned and was worse than the pain in her back.

That symptom was significant because a routine chymopapain injection shouldn't produce increased pain in the leg. Because the injection can take several days or even several weeks to produce its full benefits, and since she was suffering so much, I kept Mrs. Wilson in hospital. When there was no improvement in her condition, I ordered another CT scan to see what was going on. I was in for a surprise. Although the X-ray appearance of the spine doesn't normally change immediately after chymopapain, in this case the scan clearly showed that a portion of the lower disc had moved further into the spinal canal.

Now it was easy to see what had happened. On the fourth day after the chymopapain injection, a fragment of the nucleus, already extruding through the shell of the disc, had torn loose. Its connection to the remaining nucleus had been broken by the chemical action of the drug. Suddenly free, the piece slid down the tunnel containing the nerve root. New pressure was causing the leg pain.

As soon as I made that discovery, I knew that surgery was the only answer. I operated, found the stray piece of nucleus, and removed it easily. From the moment she came out of the anesthetic, Stacey Wilson's leg pain was gone and her back problem disappeared. After two days' rest, she went home.

And so, that one troublesome disc required surgery after all. Like most treatments chymopapain has its benefits, but it also has its limitations.

Recently I read a newspaper feature describing how some doctors are now treating back pain with injections of steroids and morphine, and having incredible success. Is this a breakthrough?

I'm afraid not. This is one of those treatments that pop up in the news every so often, and sometimes an overenthusiastic reporter will convey the impression that it's a miraculous new cure. Usually the news reports don't make the distinction between long-term benefit and temporary pain relief, and they are vague about the kind of back problem that can be helped. In this case, the treatment is aimed only at providing temporary pain relief for patients with severe symptoms after back surgery has failed. Certainly the injection provides no cure, miraculous or otherwise.

Still, it's a fairly simple procedure. Morphine, mixed with a steroid preparation, is injected into the epidural space, the space between the bony walls of the spinal canal and the fluid-filled sac around the nerves. The relief it provides is occasionally quite dramatic, although no one knows exactly why. The morphine may have some sort of general effect on the pain mechanism, or it may react locally with the coverings of the nerves. The steroid reduces any local inflammation and counteracts the irritation caused by the morphine.

The same article also mentioned other drugs that were said to be a successful means of reducing inflammation. Are these the ones you told me about before?

Yes. They're commonly called NSAIDs, which stands for non-steroidal anti-inflammatory drugs. As you know, inflammation is the body's normal reaction to injury. It results from the rapid collection of certain blood cells, specific enzymes, and various chemicals needed to heal the original damage. But an inflammatory reaction that is too strong can cause pain, so that the "cure" becomes the cause. Anti-inflammatory drugs slow this reaction down to a more or less normal pace and give an unnecessarily inflamed area a chance to recover.

That sounds like a good treatment, but from what you've said I suppose there are side effects.

You're right. In fact anti-inflammatories produce several side effects. One problem is that NSAIDs don't act just on the inflammation you want to treat – the swelling and pain in a worn spinal joint, for example; they also slow down the same reaction everywhere else in the body. In the stomach, that slowdown can cause an ulcer or serious bleeding. To protect itself against the acids and other digestive juices it contains, the stomach is continually replacing its lining cells at a rapid rate. An anti-inflammatory drug, unable to distinguish between the increased activity of inflammation and the normally speedy turnover of stomach-lining cells, will slow down both processes.

The NSAIDs can have other side effects. Some can cause headaches, skin rashes, or an unwanted retention of fluid. One type has even been known to produce acute psychotic episodes. Rarely, NSAIDs will depress the action of blood-forming tissue in the bone marrow and elsewhere, which can lead to a serious shortage of vital blood cells.

Most important of all, the non-steroidal anti-inflammatory drugs don't always solve the problem. For low-back pain they are effective only about half the time. And even when they work they must be regarded as a temporary measure to control the symptoms until natural healing can occur.

All in all, I am not enthusiastic about anti-inflammatories for low-back disorders. I prescribe them occasionally but usually as a secondary measure in the control of an acute attack already being treated with rest, counter-irritants, and gentle stretching.

A friend suggested I try acupuncture to cure my back. What do you think?

Acupuncture is a legitimate method of pain relief, but don't count on it as a sure thing, and don't think of it as a cure. According to the most reliable data I have seen, only about one-third of the people who receive acupuncture to relieve chronic back or neck pain find it effective. In some cases, the benefits seem to last a long time – for months or even for years; in other cases, the pain comes back after just a few hours or days.

Acupuncture works by somehow interfering with the normal pain-transmission system. It has no effect at all on the source or cause of the problem. The value of having tiny needles stuck in your ear, big toe, or other parts of your body to stop back pain must be weighed against the fact that sooner or later all acute attacks get better anyway and may not recur for years.

One problem with a treatment as poorly understood as acupuncture is that it breeds fads that make no scientific sense. For example, some of its practitioners have moved on to a thing called "laser acupuncture." You may know that lasers are modified beams of light that can produce enough heat to melt a brick, or be used to send signals over long distances because they travel in thin, perfectly straight lines. Neither of those properties has anything to do with acupuncture, but some people are receiving treatments with a "cold-laser probe" attached by a cord to a machine that emits an ominous hum. The whole process smacks more of Hollywood hoke than of modern medicine.

But, having stated those reservations, I'd say that if you're looking for pain relief, and conventional acupuncture appeals to you, go ahead and try it. It's harmless, and it just might help.

Is there a relationship between acupuncture and a treatment called "trigger-point therapy"?

Yes, in a way, there is. As the name implies, treatment is directed at "trigger points," small, tender lumps that sometimes mysteriously appear near the surface of the skin, usually along the tops of the shoulders or over the back of the pelvis. No one knows what causes these trigger points or even exactly what they are. They are impossible to remove surgically; they just disappear when you get under the skin. Trigger points often mark the location of pain referred from somewhere else – the neck pain you feel between your shoulder blades, for example – and these points themselves can become major sources of discomfort. But pressing on them, massaging them, or subjecting them to friction by rubbing on them rapidly, can reduce the pain they cause. Injecting them with local anesthetic is effective, and so is inserting an acupuncture needle. Many of the typical sites for these lumps correspond to the classic acupuncture points. For this reason, some practitioners believe that treating the trigger points can be beneficial to the distant site of trouble, although this two-way-street effect has never been proven to exist.

When the trigger points are widespread, with tender areas over the breast bone and at the elbows and knees as well as in the shoulders and back, the condition is often called fibrositis or tissue tension pain. Along with changes in behavior, insomnia, loss of libido, and all the other symptoms we discussed earlier, the development of numerous trigger points may accompany the chronic pain syndrome.

What about the electrical device known as a TENS unit – does it act something like acupuncture?

Sort of. TENS, or transcutaneous electrical nerve stimulation, can be an effective means of temporarily blocking unwanted pain signals. Like acupuncture, it produces a reaction that seems to liberate endorphins, naturally produced opiates that interfere with the normal transmission of pain through the upper spinal cord and the base of the brain. In the relief of some types of acute post-operative pain, TENS can reduce or even eliminate the need for other pain medication. As you might expect, the treatment has less value in chronic cases. The body can develop a resistance to the electrical stimulation, just as it can to many drugs. Consequently, a stronger and stronger input is required to produce an effect. Eventually you may reach a point where the TENS machine cannot produce an impulse sufficient to prevent the pain message from getting through. At that point the patient's symptoms will return.

On a radio phone-in show I heard a back specialist talking about thermological pain studies. Are they something new?

The term "thermological pain studies" is a fancy way of saying "thermograms," and they have been around for quite a while. Thermograms can be produced by expensive electronic techniques or, much more commonly, by latex sheets embedded with crystals that change color at various temperatures. These sheets are placed on your body and photographed to measure the temperature of your skin at various locations. That measurement, in turn, provides useful information as to the amount of blood flowing in or near the skin at that point on your body. Inflammation of the skin from any injury will produce a "hot" thermogram. So will the increased circulation in actively contracting muscles just beneath the surface.

You may have seen a thermographic study demonstrated on television. In one commercial for an aftershave lotion, viewers are shown a thermogram of a man's face right after he finishes shaving. The skin on his face records a high temperature, demonstrated by the color of the thermogram indicating an increased blood flow – which is hardly surprising, since he has just been scratching it with a razor. Then the man slaps on the aftershave and the thermogram instantly shows a remarkable change. The alcohol in the solution rapidly constricts the local blood vessels and lowers the skin temperature.

And that's all there is, really, to those "thermological pain studies" you asked about. A thermogram is a measure of local blood supply and temperature. It has some use in assessing blood flow to the limbs in vascular problems, but because it is completely non-specific a thermogram is of no diagnostic value for back complaints and it certainly does not measure pain. As a colleague of mine is fond of saying, "The most dramatic thermogram you will ever see is the picture of a blush."

I've thought of looking into a treatment called biofeedback, which is said to produce good results for backache victims. What do you think?

Biofeedback is based on your ability to exert conscious control over some of the functions of your body that are ordinarily automatic. To most people hearing about it for the first time, it sounds almost mystical. And, considering its potential for being sold as some sort of magic, I give a lot of credit to its practitioners. With rare exceptions, they are conscientious about avoiding the use of exaggerated claims or scientific doubletalk.

As a means of controlling backache, biofeedback concentrates on muscle spasm. Basically, the technique consists of recognizing that your muscles are tense, and then consciously relaxing them. During the early learning stage, you may use electrodes and meters to guide you in monitoring your responses. Once you have learned the technique, you can put the hardware aside and practice biofeedback all by yourself.

Like any other treatment, though, it has its limitations. Not everyone can master biofeedback fully, and even those who do master it cannot always apply it effectively enough to relieve a muscle spasm. Also, as you might suppose, biofeedback is a lot less useful if the chronic pain syndrome has taken hold.

In short, I offer the same advice about it as I do for acupuncture: it's harmless, and worth trying as long as your expectations are realistic. And there's a bonus in this case: if you can master it, you'll be armed with an anti-pain weapon you can use on your own, without any expense or need for medical supervision. Just remember, though, that we're talking, at most, about relieving pain – not about applying a remedy for the cause of the back problem.

Would you say the same thing about hypnosis as a means of pain relief?

That depends. If you believe hypnosis is likely to help you, it might be worth trying, provided that your doctor has assured you that your problem is primarily a matter of pain control and not something that requires direct physical treatment. I have referred patients for hypnosis on occasions when the patients themselves requested it, but I have not been impressed with the results. The idea is to change the patient's attitude, in two stages: using hypnosis first as a blocking mechanism to shut off the pain, and second as a method of motivating the patient. The pain-blocking effect works but doesn't last long, and the process of improving motivation involves functions too complex to be handled effectively by anything as simple as hypnosis. I'm prepared to believe there have been situations where hypnosis was remarkably effective, but I have never seen one.

But again, my basic rule remains the same. Alternative forms of treatment are fine if they are helpful, harmless, and unlikely to interfere with correct medical management.

A friend of mine had an operation called a "rhizolysis." Would you explain what that actually involves?

Rhizolysis or rhizotomy, as it is often called, means the deliberate destruction of the nerve supply to the small facet joints of the spine. When these joints are left without feeling, the pain from Type One problems should be eliminated.

There's nothing wrong with the theory of joint denervation, but the practice falls short. In the earliest rhizotomies the nerves were cut with a surgical scalpel, but this technique was difficult and often failed to do the job. Now rhizolysis uses a radio frequency probe that actually burns the nerves. Multiple lesions are required, since each joint may have two or even three separate nerves running to it. The problem is that it's difficult to destroy all the sensation, and even when the nerve destruction is complete, the joint can develop a new supply, allowing feeling and pain to return. Overall, for the treatment of chronic low-back pain, rhizotomy is successful in about 30 percent of patients. It is of no value in relieving Type Two, Three, or Four pain. There are risks, such as infection, related to the minor surgery. They aren't great but they must be weighed against the potential benefits of the technique.

What is your opinion of holistic medicine?

Holistic medicine is good medicine but I object to the way it is presented. Its practitioners and enthusiasts imply that no other doctors pay attention to their patients as a whole. The rest of us are accused of merely treating specific complaints as though they were isolated from the rest of the human being. This is quite untrue.

A good orthopedic surgeon, for example, will not just examine a fractured thigh bone and ignore the patient's general health. By the same token, giving that patient proper holistic treatment certainly does not mean just making him feel good and checking on his nutrition and bowel habits without paying specific attention to the broken leg. Obviously a good doctor will attend to the patient's specific problem and to his overall needs as well. Practitioners who present themselves as specialists in holistic medicine have no monopoly on good medical care.

Then you have no objection to the holistic approach?

Not when it simply represents good medicine. But I believe some of its practitioners are carrying the approach to extremes. Like many another well-meaning idea that becomes a fad, the concept of holistic medicine has been distorted by proponents who have lost the original perspective.

As a concept it took shape in reaction to increasing specialization. When the family doctor began to recede from the scene, a feeling developed that instead of going to a whole array of specialists, the patient should see one doctor who is interested in every problem. And who can argue with that? If you went to see your family doctor, I'm sure you'd want a comprehensive physical examination as well as a chance to talk not only about your head cold or your backache but also about your kids and how they're doing at school, and about your job, especially if you're having a lot of trouble at work. That's the sort of approach holistic medicine is supposed to take. The holistic practitioner is supposed to be the epitome of the good family physician.

Yet if that's all there were to holistic medicine, there would be no reason for it to exist as a separate entity, because that approach is exactly what you can expect from a competent family doctor. I think that's why holistic doctors, generally speaking, have moved away from that perfectly sensible position – so that their services will sound completely different from those of an ordinary general practitioner.

But how have they managed to sell holistic medicine as something different, if good family doctors were taking the same approach all along?

I believe a couple of other trends have helped make holistic medicine possible. One trend has been for patients to go to specialists directly, whenever they can. If you have only a bad back you probably don't want to spend time talking to your family doctor about it, because you don't believe a general practitioner knows all that much about back problems and will probably send you to someone else anyway.

As a result, people are swarming into specialists' offices with complaints that are often self-diagnosed and may or may not be accurate. Even if the complaint is not serious, most patients would rather hear that from the specialist, not from the family doctor. This trend, of course, defeats the system. The specialist sees a lot of patients who do not require his expertise, and those who do need him find it harder to get appointments.

The second trend has arisen from the first: as patients perceive that the specialist knows more about specific complaints than the general practitioner does, the family doctor comes to believe the same thing. If the doctor is told often enough that the public, as represented by his patients, is not interested in his opinion on, say, bad backs, then he stops offering his opinion. And so he abdicates the responsibility, no longer attempting to keep up to date on back care. Ironically, then, the family physician actually helps fill the system with patients referred unnecessarily to specialists.

At this point, the holistic medicine man, with the same medical training as the family doctor, enters the picture, presenting himself as a specialist. He is, so to speak, a "specialist in general practice." And whereas the family doctor may be seen as only a GP – a sort of medical jack-of-all-trades – the holistic doctor is a "specialist" specializing in everything.

Now, if he is to justify that claim, the holistic practitioner must develop special techniques. He must do things the average family physician can't do, so as to give his work a special mystique or at least an air of specialization involving knowledge beyond what you'd expect of your average doctor.

And so we find holistic medicine offering such rarefied services as hair analysis, which purports to look for trace mineral losses indicative of the body's needs. The technique has no scientific validity, and in fact a lab analysis of the same hair sample will not usually produce the same results twice. This is one reason why hair analysis is looked upon with great suspicion by all reputable scientific bodies.

That brings us to one of the great ironies of holistic medicine. Many of its practitioners provide some sort of special diagnostic technique, such as hair analysis, at the same time claiming to treat the patient as a unique organism, and then turn around and prescribe exactly the same treatment as they've prescribed for virtually all their other patients – vitamins, well-balanced diets, and proper living habits, all the common-sense things you were taught back in high school health classes.

But at least holistic medicine is harmless.

Not necessarily. Suppose you have something seriously wrong with you that hasn't been diagnosed. With the array of physical, radio-logical, and laboratory investigations currently available, it makes no sense to rely almost exclusively on a single test, particularly one so questionable as hair analysis. And yet a holistic practitioner may complete only a chemical diagnosis and then proceed to treat you with vitamin supplements and minerals, without paying much attention to the other aspects of the problem. At that point, holistic medicine, in my view, becomes dangerous, and the term "holistic" itself becomes ironically inappropriate.

What about some of the other alternative approaches – craniosacral therapy, for example?

Craniosacral therapy is based on several fascinating and totally unproven concepts. One deals with the transfer of a kind of "body electricity" from the therapist to the patient. Another describes a "natural pulse" within the central nervous system that can supposedly be felt through a periodic enlargement of the skull and an associated upward movement of the sacrum. What this theory seems to be saying is that your body behaves something like one of those instant toy poodles that entertainers construct out of balloons at children's parties: if you squeeze the air-filled poodle's mid-section his head grows bigger, and vice versa. That's more or less what the craniosacral people believe happens to your spine and head: six to twelve times a minute your spine grows shorter and your head gets larger; then your head shrinks and your spine elongates.

Proponents of craniosacral therapy also see it as a modern application of the classic yoga theory of "superphysical filaments" which, if they exist at all, have so far eluded discovery by medical science. Craniosacralists link the concept to the martial arts, therapeutic touch, and the widely publicized "Philippine psychic surgery," in which the healer appears to reach inside the sufferer's body with his bare hands and yet not leave a mark on the skin.

The scientific basis for craniosacral therapy rests on theories originally put forward by an osteopathic student in the early 1900s. Although anatomic studies showed, then as now, that the bones of the adult skull are incapable of independent movement, he felt that since joint lines were visible and since all of nature's designs have a purpose, movement must take place.

Today, craniosacral therapy exists as a manipulative technique to adjust the immovable bones in the adult cranium and to take advantage of the body's natural rhythm and the normal "direction of energy." It has never been proven to have any benefit over conventional forms of manipulation. Certainly the concept of diagnosing and treating spinal problems by perceiving and altering the expansion and contraction of the skull is well beyond the fringe of accepted medical practice.

I never dreamed that writing a book on back pain would lead me into a discussion of shrunken heads, but there you are.

What about some of the more widely accepted sources of treatment – osteopaths, for instance?

Osteopathy is a respectable and valuable profession, and I have no objection to my patients' seeing one of its practitioners, if that's what they want. Of course, I want to be sure their condition will be diagnosed properly before any treatment is undertaken.

Are osteopaths qualified to diagnose most back problems?

Yes, they are. In training and professional qualifications, an osteopath is closer to a doctor than to a chiropractor. As most people know, someone wanting to become a doctor must obtain a university degree, then attend a recognized medical school, usually in a four-year program. After that comes a year of internship, roughly equivalent to an apprenticeship. Additional training is required for a doctor to qualify as a specialist.

Generally, the educational requirements to become a doctor of osteopathy (DO), are much the same as those for becoming an MD, except, of course, that the students attend a school of osteopathy instead of a medical school. Since "osteo" means bone, you might assume that an osteopath treats only bone conditions. But in the United States, osteopaths, while concentrating particularly on manipulative therapy, are trained and licensed to perform the same services as general practitioners, and they treat such non-skeletal conditions as diabetes and high blood pressure. With extra training, they can even perform surgery.

In other countries there are differing restrictions on the services osteopaths are allowed to perform. In most Canadian provinces, osteopaths are licensed as chiropractors and are allowed to provide only chiropractic-type drugless therapy. An osteopath practicing as a chiropractor can manipulate or "adjust" your spinal joints and may administer physical treatments such as hot packs and whirlpool baths. But he is allowed to offer you only non-prescription medication such as vitamin pills.

Chiropractors have a narrower range of medical knowledge and diagnostic skills than DOs or MDs. They are trained specifically to deal with problems that can be resolved by manipulation. Typically, they are required to complete two years of university before entering a four-year course at chiropractic college, where their studies concentrate largely on spinal anatomy and manipulation of the spine. Successful students emerge with a Doctor of Chiropractic (DC) degree.

Many doctors are sharply critical of chiropractors. Where do you stand?

I have no quarrel with the treatments most chiropractors give back-pain sufferers. But I think it's important for you, as the patient, to realize that the "adjustments" a chiropractor makes to your spine have no long-term benefits. If they did, you wouldn't have to keep going for chiropractic treatments month after month or year after year. It is quite possible that a chiropractor will relieve a muscle spasm that is causing you back pain. And there's nothing wrong with that. But if you want to prevent the problem from recurring, you need to follow a long-term maintenance program that will yield long-term benefits. And that's not something you can hope to get from repeated manipulation.

Patients sometimes tell me, "I've been going to my chiropractor for the past ten [or whatever] years."

I ask: "Has he helped you to get rid of your back pain?"

"No."

"Then why do you go back to him?"

"Because he does me a lot of good."

The chiropractic profession thrives on that kind of doublethink. There aren't many patients these days who would stay with the same doctor for ten years, waiting for him to solve the original problem.

Is that why doctors often criticize chiropractors – because their treatments offer only short-term relief and have to be repeated indefinitely?

That may be one reason. But I think most doctors take exception not to what the chiropractor *does* but to what he *says* he does. Chiropractors often talk about discs and joints that have "gone out of place." Yet, as you know by now, discs don't slip and joints don't routinely "go in and out of place."

Your sore back can feel stiff and strange, but that doesn't mean the joints are out of place. And why should you assume they are? After all, when you sprain your thumb, you don't automatically assume that the joint has "gone out." So why should you think anything different about the joints in your spine? Believe me, they are encased far more securely than your thumb joints.

But I'm sure I've felt and heard my back go out – it made a cracking sound.

What you heard is essentially the same thing you hear when people crack their knuckles. The joints in your fingers and in your spine contain nitrogen dissolved under pressure in a small amount of joint fluid. If you decrease the pressure – by pulling on your fingers and enlarging the joint space, for instance – the nitrogen comes out of solution and turns into gas, going "pop" just the way a bottle of champagne pops when you uncork it. But whether the joint is in a finger or your spine, nothing has gone out of place when it "cracks." Yet some chiropractors will encourage you to believe otherwise. Just ask yourself: when was the last time you saw anyone rearrange his fingers just by cracking his knuckles?

Chiropractors have a whole lexicon of terms they love to toss around. I find that as objectionable as speaking Doctor when plain English will do. I know one woman whose chiropractor told her that her neck had lost its "motoricity." Now there's a piece of jargon for the auto-makers in Detroit to conjure with! ("Test drive the Zoomjet 88 – it's tops in motoricity!") And just in case he hadn't frightened the poor woman enough with that one, the chiropractor also told her she suffered from "multiple subluxation complexes."

But I don't think that's all just chiropractic jargon. I'm sure I've heard my own doctor use some of those words.

You're right. It's not just chiropractic jargon; it's also medical jargon. Luxation means dislocation, and subluxation therefore means "something less than a complete dislocation." Never mind the accuracy of the diagnosis; let's deal just with the jargon. Since there is no single English word that precisely means "subluxation," I give the chiropractor full marks for precision in the use of the term, even though the patient couldn't understand what he said. However, when he spoke of "multiple subluxation complexes" he was talking pretentious nonsense. "Multiple" just means many or several, and "complexes," in that context, doesn't mean anything at all. In my view, if a doctor or chiropractor tries to impress his patients with mumbo jumbo like that, he probably doesn't have much else to offer.

Some people are convinced that many doctors are jealous of chiropractors.

I wouldn't say jealous, but doctors may well envy chiropractors for developing such strong loyalty in their patients. Much as they would like to, few doctors can evoke that kind of response. One reason is that doctors, particularly specialists, usually treat patients for a limited period of time, and if the treatment is successful they don't arrange to see them again. Chiropractors, on the other hand, tend to require frequent follow-up or maintenance visits, regardless of whether the patient still has trouble. That continuing contact often creates a bond.

But there are other reasons as well. A past president of the American Chiropractic Association told me that chiropractors were kept busy treating patients with back problems partly because doctors had abdicated their responsibility. He said most MDs were not interested in treating backs and were happy to let somebody else take over. I think there is a great deal of truth in that. A doctor who shows little concern for the patients' problems can hardly expect loyalty from them.

Also, because of their broader knowledge and the caution typical of the profession, many doctors may hesitate or worry aloud over the correct diagnosis and treatment of a back problem. Their apparent indecision raises the patient's concerns that the problem is more serious, or at least more difficult, than he or she expected. Most chiropractors are far more decisive. They'll say to the patient, "I know exactly what's wrong and how to make it right. Now if you'll just lie down here on this table...."

That's what people want to hear when they're bewildered and frightened about a medical problem. It gives them hope and confidence in their ability to get better. And that's an important step towards recovery regardless of who initiates it. Once he's got that going for him, it may not even matter whether the chiropractor's physical manipulation is effective.

But every time I get treated at the chiropractor's I come out feeling good. Are you saying that manipulation isn't really helping me?

No, that's not what I'm saying. If you have pain when you go in and it's gone when you come out, you are obviously gaining some benefit. Like any other valid form of therapy, manipulation can produce desirable results if it is applied properly and in the right circumstances. But remember, it's not a cure, and if you visit your chiropractor even when you have no pain – perhaps because you made the appointment well in advance and because you know you'll feel good afterwards – you ought to ask yourself what's really going on. Is the visit simply an indulgence, on a par with a leisurely soak in the bathtub? Are you beginning to rely on treatments you don't really need? And, if so, to what extent is your chiropractor actively encouraging you to become dependent on him?

But can't I trust a professional to make the proper decisions?

This is not a matter of trust but a matter of *responsibility*. It's your back we're talking about here, and the primary responsibility for looking after it belongs to you, no matter what specialists you see or how trustworthy they are. You are the one who must make the important distinction between a treatment that really helps your back get better and one that merely makes you "feel good."

One example of a "feel good" treatment is massage. Even from a registered therapist, massage is just another way of gaining muscle relaxation. It has no lasting effect. But if you are tense and suffer from muscle tension pain, a vigorous massage can certainly make you feel better. The problem is that patients may become dependent on these treatments, which require no active participation and provide only short-term comfort. The treatments become a means of avoiding the responsibility of taking charge.

What's the difference between a chiropractic adjustment and the manipulation I might receive from a physical therapist?

Basically there is no difference. "Adjustment" is simply the chiropractor's term for manipulation. Applied to the spine, manipulation means putting your back joints through a range of movement. Whether manipulation is done quickly or slowly, forcefully or gently, to the whole spine or part of it, and whether the range of movement is part of, all of, or slightly more than the joint's normal capability depends on the practitioner and the circumstances. No matter which kind of specialist performs the manipulation – a chiropractor, an osteopath, a physical therapist, or an MD – it's essentially the same thing.

You've mentioned training for osteopaths and chiropractors. What about physical therapists?

The physical therapist graduates from a four-year university program with a bachelor degree, though many continue training in a specialty – such as orthopedics, pediatrics, cardiovascular rehabilitation, and manipulation techniques. Masters and PhD programs in physical therapy now exist in many large universities throughout North America. The four-year course also includes a clinical internship with considerable practical exposure.

In the typical situation, physical therapists are allowed to treat only at the direction of a doctor, and cannot accept unreferred patients. Unlike chiropractors, they must function as part of a medical team. Through this close association, I have come to appreciate their role in the physical treatment of back problems and have learned a great deal about the value of manipulative therapy.

From what you've learned, how does manipulation relieve pain?

We think the pain relief results from the release of muscle spasm or the return of normal movement to stiff spinal joints, but we don't know exactly why or how manipulation works. Even the experts can't determine whether the benefit of stretching comes from its effect on the joint lining or capsule, or the muscle sheath, or even the fat under the skin. All we can say for sure is that manipulation does relieve back pain for some people sometimes.

Studies have shown that manipulation has no long-term effect: those who are going to get better do so with it or without it. Its role seems to be to shorten the duration of the problem, and that's a good thing in itself. But if I were selling medical "cures," rather than dispensing advice, I could easily draw on my professional experience to "prove" that manipulation is the answer for common backache.

On one occasion I was supervising minor surgery when a nurse from another operating room came and asked whether she could have an appointment with me soon. She explained that she had a muscle spasm in her neck. Since I wasn't scrubbed for the operation I suggested we might just as well do something about her problem right there and then. I had her lie down on a spare table in the operating room and after I examined her I "adjusted" her neck. The manipulation immediately relieved her pain. She got up and left the room – pain free.

On another occasion a friend of mine and his wife were over

for a visit. When she complained of a pain in her low back, I offered to examine her. I decided manipulation might help, so I had her lie down on a table and I proceeded to manipulate her back. It was another one of those treatments that provided instant relief.

That's just the way things go, sometimes, with manipulation. Since it took only a few minutes, and neither woman was really expecting much change, if the manipulation hadn't succeeded they probably would have quickly written off the experience as just another treatment that didn't happen to work. As it was, they were delighted with the result and may well have told others about my skill.

Chiropractors thrive on that kind of selective, word-of-mouth publicity, and who can blame them? But even their successes prove nothing about the validity of chiropractic theory.

But you'd have to admit that to most patients, theory doesn't matter a lot – it's results that count.

That's usually how patients feel, and I don't blame them. Manipulation has its place, and as long as it is preceded by proper diagnosis, so there is no question about the cause of the problem and the safety of the "adjustments," I don't object to that form of therapy for anyone who wants to try it. I frequently refer patients for manipulation, usually to a specially trained physical therapist and occasionally to a chiropractor. Your chances of being helped temporarily are better than fifty-fifty, and you might turn out to be one of the lucky ones.

However, I'm thinking more generally about alternative forms of treatment when I say it's a mistake to ignore theory and simply ask whether a treatment produces results. A lot of questionable procedures have been sold to desperate people on the basis of a few good results, which may or may not be indicative of the soundness and value of the technique. In some instances, the practitioners impress prospective patients by citing testimonials from well-known doctors, medical institutions, or recognized medical journals. It all sounds very convincing and few doctors or patients ever have the time and inclination to check out the references.

Not long ago, I was asked to comment on the value of a treatment called prolotherapy, which involves injecting various fluids into the spine to "tighten up the ligaments." The whole theory is highly questionable, but that's not central to the point I'm making here. Prolotherapy, which first surfaced about thirty years ago, had recently been taken up by a local family doctor who obviously seemed to believe in it and wanted the Workers' Compensation Board to approve and pay for it. When the board refused and the doctor concerned persisted, I was asked for an opinion, and so I looked into the claims he was making.

In one of his letters, the doctor had said the value of the treatment was mentioned in a well-known orthopedic textbook. He even cited the edition and relevant page numbers. So I got a copy of the book. I found that either this doctor hadn't read the text carefully, or he'd assumed that nobody would bother to look up the reference. In fact, what the author had written about prolotherapy injections was disturbing news for the doctor and his patients.

The book cited two reports published in the *Journal of the American Medical Association*, which described two prolotherapy cases that turned out badly. One patient ended up as a spastic paraplegic and the other developed serious symptoms and then died following surgery undertaken to relieve them. The author also related first-hand experiences with patients sent to him after prolotherapy. He said he couldn't see any benefit from the injections, and that his "overall personal opinion of the technique" was "not favorable."

So much for documented references offered as "proof" that a treatment is valid. Even if the sources cited actually support the claims being made for a treatment, there may also be any number of unfavorable reports that are intentionally left unmentioned.

But what if the supportive statement has come from a highly qualified doctor whose credentials are beyond question?

You won't often find highly accredited medical specialists making declarations of that kind in support of any radically new treatment. But even if they do they can still be wrong. They may have been misled by incomplete or erroneous information, or they may be basing their statements on a sampling that was too small to be conclusive.

I realize that, as a group, doctors are regarded as arch conservatives when it comes to accepting new techniques. Some people would carry that criticism even further; they are willing to believe that superior discoveries and new treatments are continually being suppressed by the medical establishment to avoid embarrassment or the loss of income that would ensue if established procedures had to be abandoned.

That "conspiracy" theory, of course, ignores the fact that there are scores of medicines, machines, and techniques in use today that were unheard of even five or ten years ago. Certainly the establishment has no vested interest in keeping you sick – least of all if you have a bad back. Most doctors would be delighted to find a way of eliminating back pain. General practitioners don't like treating it because of the uncertainties and frustrations involved; and most orthopedic surgeons, myself included, would welcome the chance to devote more time to patients with injuries or other problems.

Meanwhile, before you try any "revolutionary cure" or "new natural therapy as seen on TV," you and your doctor should scrutinize it carefully to determine its real value and possible drawbacks. Since your own back will be the test site, would you really want to do anything less?

11. TOOLS OF THE BACK DOCTOR'S TRADE

Every so often, a patient of mine describes some feeling or observation so perfectly that I feel compelled to record it and find a place to use it in my lectures or my writing.

One of those memorable observations came from a woman who shares my enthusiasm for analogies. She told me a story that precisely described the problem of her back pain, which was defying my best efforts at diagnosis and treatment.

Her husband, an automobile mechanic, had gone to work on their own car because it was stalling frequently. He checked every possible cause, or so he thought, and replaced several parts in case they were faulty. But the stalling persisted, occurring at unpredictable intervals. Everything he did made the car run a little better but never really solved the problem.

Finally, after deducing that the trouble had to be somewhere in the gas line, he spotted a tiny thread near the end of the pipe. That was the clue he needed: a fragment of cloth, probably from a previous maintenance job, was loose in the pipe and was intermittently blocking the flow of gasoline.

And, as my patient observed, "Isn't that something like my back trouble? It comes and it goes, and there are a lot of things you are doing for me – getting me to exercise and practice good back care and lose weight – and those things are all helping a little. But you've never really gotten to the source of the problem – the real thing that makes my back hurt."

With that fitting analogy, she announced her discovery of an inevitable truth about back problems: although we have many remedies to try, they are never fully successful unless we are treating the right problem.

However, we *are* solving more and more of those diagnostic riddles, thanks to modern technology.

At a recent meeting in San Francisco, a colleague of mine declared that in his practice the CT scan has already replaced physical examination of the back. I think that's an overestimation of the machine's capabilities. It's like saying that once people can shop by closed-circuit television they will never want to enter a store again. But there are just some things a picture can't tell you about that sofa you're thinking of buying. Don't you want to bounce on the cushions and feel the texture and personally examine the workmanship?

Diagnosing back problems involves many aspects that shouldn't be left to a machine, and I don't believe that current technology can provide a substitute for the human perceptions and insights that so often make the difference in a difficult diagnosis.

And yet I certainly share my colleague's enthusiasm for the modern medical tools which have become invaluable aids to suggest and confirm the diagnoses made by traditional means. This chapter explains why.

X-rays are used routinely for back trouble. Aren't they actually quite dangerous?

Not really. Unfortunately, most people have an anxiety about X-rays that has no basis in present-day reality. Their fears may be based on stories from the early days of X-ray work when researchers had their fingers burned off because they had no idea there was any danger, or on frightening descriptions of the effects that follow an atomic explosion. There is a growing concern about the cumulative effect of low-level radiation. And, of course, there are the numerous exposés written by consumer advocates "piercing the veil of medical secrecy" and detailing "the horrors of excessive X-ray exposure."

The resulting public reaction to X-rays reminds me of an experience I had not long ago, when my colleagues and I treated an unusual illness in a recent immigrant to our country. It turned out to be a case of leprosy – not a disease you expect to find in most hospitals in the western world. Some of the other doctors were aghast at the diagnosis, and I would probably have reacted the same way if I hadn't worked for a time in the Far East, where I became accustomed to seeing perhaps three or four cases of leprosy a month. From that experience I came to appreciate that leprosy is a treatable disease with a remarkably low rate of contagion. Doctors can work among lepers for years and never contract leprosy themselves.

Everyone trained in modern medicine may know these facts intellectually, and yet there were a few of my well-educated contemporaries who reacted much the way people did in biblical times, when anyone suspected of having leprosy was not permitted to walk through a village without crying out the warning, "Unclean! Unclean!"

Many people harbor a similarly uninformed fear of X-rays. They associate them with such horrors as genetic mutations brought on by radiation poisoning. And X-ray technologists, intent on reassuring patients that no harm will come to them, take elaborate precautions to protect themselves with leaded shields and aprons, thereby unintentionally reinforcing those already exaggerated fears. No one may bother to point out that while the patient will be exposed to half a dozen X-rays that day, the technicians will have the potential for being exposed to several hundred that day and every other working day of their lives.

X-rays, in short, are not nearly as dangerous as most people believe. But there is clearly another side to the story. Some doctors and chiropractors suggest or even insist on obtaining radiographs when there is little or no indication that they will be of value. A patient of mine was seen in the emergency room of a local hospital for an acute attack of neck and shoulder pain. The record I saw later described her symptoms clearly as a typical acute attack of local muscle spasm with no nerve involvement. In spite of the simple and obvious diagnosis, no one in Emergency would treat her without seeing an X-ray. My patient really felt forced into submitting to a series of cervical spine films, which, of course, showed nothing abnormal.

Usually the X-ray's diagnostic value far outweighs the minimal risk of exposure. But charging an extra fee for unnecessary radiological tests, or getting an X-ray as a substitute for good clinical judgment, or as protection against a possible malpractice action, is unfair to the patient. The small amount of extra radiation may not be harmful, but it isn't good for you, either.

I wouldn't make such a point of discussing the balance between the proper role and the misuse of X-ray if popular misconceptions didn't interfere with the care I try to provide. I have had patients tell me they were unwilling to undergo necessary X-rays or a CT scan to assist the diagnosis of their orthopedic problem because they had already had "too much radiation" from routine chest X-rays. Such concerns are groundless. The amount of radiation you get during a routine chest film is negligible, and the amount to which you are exposed during a properly controlled CT study is not much more.

Radiologists themselves have inadvertently fed this fear by setting extremely conservative standards for exposure. When they assure people it's safe to have, say, one X-ray every six months, the implication is that it would be unsafe to have four or five X-rays a year, when in fact even at that rate, your exposure would be far below the slightest degree of danger.

I have heard people talk about EMG machines. Are they a form of X-ray?

No, EMG stands for electromyography, which is the study of how a muscle reacts when it is stimulated by its nerve. Your doctor might want to study your muscle reaction if, for instance, you have back pain and have lost the ability to lift your toes while your foot is flat on the floor. To conduct the test, the examiner will insert extremely fine needles into various muscles in your leg. The needles, which you'll find uncomfortable but not painful, are connected to an instrument that reads the electrical pattern caused by contraction of the muscle. A skilled EMG interpretation can tell the doctor whether there is muscle damage or a lack of nerve stimulus, and whether that is a new, progressing problem, an old recovering problem, or a chronic, unchanging one.

The same equipment can also study the ability of the nerve itself to conduct impulses. The needles are inserted in much the same way as for the study of muscle reaction, but in this case, the instrument is used to measure the velocity of the message or impulse traveling through the nerve from one muscle group to the next. If the impulse takes longer than normal to travel a given distance, we know there is a block within the nerve.

This test is quite useful in some parts of the body but less so near the spine, because we can't obtain measurements on both sides of the point where we suspect the nerve is being pinched. Still, the test can be used to rule out blockages at other locations along the rest of the nerve, so that we can conclude, by deduction, that the problem must be in the nerve root as it leaves the vertebral column.

Are EMGs an important diagnostic tool for back specialists?

Some doctors in my field consider EMGs very useful; others regard them as a waste of time. Generally, I've found that an EMG will not give me more information than I can get from a good clinical examination. Occasionally, though, I have made clinical judgments which changed following electromyography. For instance, I've had cases where muscle weakness was present in both legs or both arms but where one side was so much weaker than the other I concluded that only one side was involved. But when the EMG studies clearly demonstrated abnormal muscle reactions on both sides, they significantly altered my opinion. In situations like that I have learned to appreciate the value of the EMG.

Do you really need a high-tech machine like that to measure nerve function? I'm pretty sure an aunt of mine was tested simply with an anesthetic injection into the nerve.

That's not quite the same test. A nerve-root injection is done with local anesthetic to temporarily deaden the nerve the way a dentist does before he drills your teeth. In some patients it is difficult to tell which nerve root is causing pain, and freezing the roots one after another is a way to find out. When the injection stops the pain, we assume we have found the nerve carrying the message. Of course that only tells us where the trouble is, not what is causing it.

The same type of test is done by injecting the facet joints. In cases of Type One pain, anesthetizing the small spinal joints may help to localize the problem.

Both these procedures are designed to relieve back pain temporarily. In that respect they are the opposite of a discogram, which is intended to increase your pain briefly, for diagnostic purposes.

Are a myelogram and a discogram just different names for the same thing?

Not at all, but there are similarities. They are diagnostic procedures that are usually undertaken as preludes to surgery, and both are based on the same principle: the injection of a radiopaque fluid – that is, a fluid that completely blocks the penetration of the X-ray beam.

How are those injections helpful?

When the patient is X-rayed the fluid will appear white because the material completely prevents exposure of the photographic plate by the X-rays. The shape assumed by the contrast material within the body will outline structures not normally seen by X-ray – such as a bulging disc. This sort of image tells doctors more about a spinal condition than they could discover from a plain X-ray alone.

Then what's the difference between the two kinds of "grams"?

In the myelogram, the material is injected into the dural sac. This is the fluid-filled sheath that surrounds the spinal cord and the nerve roots. In the discogram, the material is injected into the disc itself.

What would make a doctor choose one instead of the other?

The myelogram gives the doctor information about the condition of the nerve sac. A tumor growing on a nerve, for instance, would block the flow of the injected material and show up as a defect on the X-ray picture. Similarly, pressure from outside the sac from a bulging disc or bony narrowing of the canal might impede the progress of the fluid and be seen on the X-ray. Determining whether the obstruction is inside or outside the dural sac requires a lot of experience in reading myelograms. And, keep in mind, the problem can be seen only if it directly affects the dura – the membrane sleeve around the nerves – and alters the flow of the fluid.

The discogram outlines the center of the disc itself and can detect abnormalities even when there is no nerve pressure. Discograms are sometimes used to localize the site of disc pain or determine whether a disc adjacent to the one selected for surgery is normal.

Discograms can give information only about the specific level that is injected. Myelograms can screen an entire section of the spine.

Incidentally, there are two more "grams" I should mention. One is an epidural venogram. In this test the radiopaque fluid is injected into the veins that run inside the spinal canal. The idea is to observe a blockage in the normal venous flow outlining a bulging disc. The other procedure is an epidurogram, in which the fluid is injected around the dural sac, rather than inside it as in a myelogram. The test was developed to avoid possible toxic effects from the older types of contrast medium on the nerves inside the sac. The epidurogram has the same basic purpose – that is to enable the doctor to detect and study a bulging disc – but since it produces a picture that's very difficult to interpret and since the new radiopaque materials are much safer, this procedure isn't used much any more.

What do they do when they give me a myelogram?

You are asked to lie down on a tilting table. The radiologist uses a long needle to inject the fluid into your dural sac, and has the table tilted in a gentle, see-saw motion. The tilting causes the fluid to flow slowly up and down your spine, filling the space around each nerve. As this is going on, X-rays are taken from various positions. All this takes about fifteen to twenty-five minutes, depending on which kind of fluid is used. The older type is an oil-based liquid that must be removed by means of a second needle when the test is finished. That extra step adds a little time to the procedure and accounts for certain post-myelogram problems. The newer type of material is a water-soluble liquid, which rapidly disappears from the spinal fluid by itself and is eventually excreted from the body.

Is a myelogram painful?

Sometimes, but not always. Some people find it painless with only mildly uncomfortable after-effects. One patient of mine, a young woman, said she "didn't feel a thing." Another patient, a middle-aged man who considered himself "a pretty tough guy," said later that the myelogram aggravated his sore back, produced terrible neck pain, and left him with a raging headache.

Is that why you hear such horrible stories about myelograms?

Could be. But a lot of those stories are greatly exaggerated. If you believe them, you may arrive at the hospital expecting the worst and be much more likely to have an unpleasant time. The headache that sometimes follows a myelogram is usually due to a lowering of the spinal fluid pressure within the dural sac, which also surrounds the brain. Most of the liquid removed is taken out when the oil-based contrast material is extracted at the end of the procedure. The body rapidly replaces the missing fluid, and the headache disappears. Obviously, with the water-based compound this is less of a problem. Other reactions may occur because of the patient's sensitivity to the material itself or because of irritation at the site of an obstruction. But in many cases, a lot of the trouble arises from tension. Everything seems to hurt more when you are tense. If you manage to walk in relaxed and unafraid, you could be pleasantly surprised at how routine and painless the procedure can be.

How can I avoid being nervous?

A lot depends on how much you understand beforehand. Ideally, your physician will give you a good briefing in advance. But some doctors don't communicate as well as they might, and if you're already upset or anxious about the prospect of surgery, you might not be taking everything in.

The radiologist, or whoever is actually administering the test, is usually responsible for making sure you understand what the myelogram is all about. While helping you overcome any fears you may have, the radiologist should also make you understand that a myelogram is more than a quick needle and a couple of X-rays. Most radiologists I know clearly outline the procedure, discuss the possible after-effects, and mention the risks involved.

Are you saying it's a risky procedure?

Only in the sense that there's some risk involved in any invasive procedure, whether it's having your tonsils out or getting a tetanus shot. There's always a possibility, however slim, that you may develop an infection, encounter unexpected bleeding, or react in an unusual way to the injected material. But to put it in perspective: having a myelogram is far less risky than driving on a busy highway.

Does it take long to recover from a myelogram? What about the after-effects?

The after-effects vary a lot from one person to the next. If your experience is average, you will have a mild headache for a day or two. A lot depends on how carefully you obey the doctor's instructions. The usual prescribed post-myelogram routine is bed rest in the hospital for eighteen to twenty-four hours. The more you raise your head the more likely you are to feel the effects of the pressure-drop I mentioned earlier. Again, this is more of a problem with the older oil-based medium. If you've had that material injected, some doctors won't let you sit up at all, not even to take nourishment. When you want to eat or drink, all you can do is stay horizontal and roll sideways.

The routine is similar if you had the water-soluble injection, except that you don't have to lie down for as long – eight to twelve hours is average. And in this case you are instructed to lie with your head slightly raised, on two pillows, for instance. The headache after this type of myelogram comes directly from irritation by the injected material. Raising your head helps keep it out of the fluid around your brain. For many of the reasons I've mentioned, this material is rapidly replacing the older oil-based type.

Some people go home from a myelogram thinking they can

cheat on the doctor's orders. Usually they pay a price, with more severe headaches, nausea, and vomiting. Fortunately, although they may be very uncomfortable, they aren't doing themselves any lasting harm.

What happens during and after a discogram?

With the usual technique, you lie on your side while the radiologist inserts a stout needle with a removable core into your back. He views the insertion on a fluoroscope screen to make sure the position is right and then slips the core out. Now the needle serves as a guiding sleeve into which the radiologist slips a slimmer, longer needle. Once this second needle is positioned in the center of the disc he injects the radiopaque fluid.

The doctors will study two things – the behavior of the contrast material in the disc, as shown on the X-ray plates, and the change in your pain. If the X-ray shows a white blob remaining in the middle of the disc, the outer shell is probably intact. If the injected fluid can be seen leaking out, there has been a tear and the disc is considered abnormal.

More important than the X-ray appearance, however, is the pain produced by the test. As the material is injected, you are asked to report whether the pain you feel is identical (or almost identical) to the typical pain you have been having. If it is, the radiologist knows that he has found the offending disc.

That sounds like a pretty uncomfortable test.

I've never met anyone who enjoyed a discogram, but there are some consoling aspects. For one thing, the painful period is quite brief – only a couple of minutes. Also, the after-effects are generally less than those of the myelogram. It's not unusual for a patient to get up after a discogram, with no need for a recovery period.

Earlier you called myelograms and discograms "preludes to surgery."

Yes, and a colleague of mine calls them "road maps for surgery," and that is about right. These tests shouldn't be used to tell the surgeon *whether* to operate – that decision should be based on sound clinical judgment – but they can certainly find the trouble and show *where* to operate. Determining exactly which disc is causing pain, or just where the nerve root is being squeezed, leads to precise and successful surgery. Some of the newer techniques, such as the CT scan, are beginning to take the place of the "grams," but for now these contrast studies remain the standard against which other tests are measured.

You have mentioned the CT scan several times, and of course I have heard of it before, but I'm still not sure exactly what it is.

CT, or CAT, is short for computerized axial tomography. It is the image produced by an extremely sophisticated computerized X-ray machine. Tomography has been around for quite a while. The name means X-rays taken at various depths of focus. The effect is sort of like a loaf of sliced bread: one tomograph gives you a view of one slice. From these X-ray "slices" the CT scanner integrates and constructs views of the body that could never be obtained in any other way. The machine also enhances minor differences in density that the human eye alone could not detect on an X-ray plate. In other words, the CT does for the X-ray what computerized photographs have done for pictures of the planets. You have probably seen photos taken during space exploration, where computers have interpreted and enhanced what the camera saw. In the same way the CT scan allows us to see things such as nerve roots and disc bulges that are invisible on plain X-rays or conventional tomograms.

In the course of a few years the CT scan has become an invaluable tool for diagnosing certain problems in the human spine. Nowhere is this more apparent than in the assessment of spinal stenosis. The CT scan provides the surgeon with cross-sectional X-ray views of the spinal canal, showing exactly where the nerve roots are in relation to the bony sidewalls or a bulging disc. This one machine has changed our understanding of spinal stenosis and how it causes nerve-root compression. Personally, I won't operate on a patient with *cauda equina* claudication from a narrow spinal canal unless I have seen a CT scan.

Another area where the CT scan has produced dramatic results is in cases of severe spinal trauma. For the first time we are able to see the pattern of the vertebral fractures and identify fragments

of bone or disc that may have burst into the canal. With this
information, the surgeon can operate to decompress the spinal
cord or nerve roots and may be able to reduce or prevent paralysis.

In many situations, the CT scan is obviously superior to the
myelogram; but the myelogram is still used extensively, either
because a CT scan is unavailable, or because the doctor has
encountered a case where the CT image doesn't provide enough
information. However, as this technology improves and the
machine becomes more widely available, we are steadily moving
closer to the day when the CT will completely supplant the myelogram as a diagnostic tool.

I value the CT scan the way people prize their personal computers: once you have come to rely on the machine you wonder
how you ever got along without it. Certainly that was true in the
case of a policeman who came to me with an unusual complaint –
and an unhappy history of injuries. While he was working as a
traffic officer, a car collided with his motorcycle and he was thrown
onto his back. A few years later, as a mounted policeman, he
suffered a second episode of back pain while mucking out the
police stables.

Three weeks before he came to me, he suffered another low-
back attack accompanied for the first time by pain in his left leg.
After two days' rest, the pain subsided from both locations, but
he noticed his foot was slapping on the ground as he walked.
He had no power to lift the foot normally.

I knew that the weakness of ankle movement indicated nerve
damage. But my examination produced some confusing findings.
The policeman could perform sit-ups easily and without pain
(which ruled out acute disc trouble) and his straight-leg raising
caused no discomfort (which ruled out nerve irritation). But
arching the spine backwards was painful, a finding which usually
indicates facet joint pain. However, facet pain and damaged nerves
don't commonly go together. And so I had a riddle on my hands:
if the patient had only facet trouble, what was he doing with a
slapping foot caused by nerve damage?

It seemed to me there was only one possible answer. The
policeman's third attack had begun with an L_4-L_5 disc rupture.
A piece of the nucleus had blown out through the shell and
completely left the disc. It hit the L_5 nerve root hard enough
to stop the nerve from working. That would cause the foot drop,
and the sudden pressure without local inflammation wouldn't cause

the typical signs of nerve-root irritation. After the fragment broke free, the shell of the disc closed up and repaired itself, which accounted for the lack of acute disc symptoms. That piece of nucleus was left in the spinal canal to continue pressing on the nerve. And so when the patient arched backwards he not only brought the facet joints more tightly together – the usual cause of Type One pain – but he also narrowed the nerve's exit tunnel, increasing pressure from the loose chunk of disc.

That was my hypothesis, based on my examination of the policeman's back. It fitted the history and the findings exactly – but how could I be sure I was right? A few years earlier, I would have had nowhere to turn for confirmation. A routine myelogram rarely fills the nerve sleeve far enough into the root canal to show the defect caused by a fragment stuck in that location. Now I simply ordered a CT scan and, sure enough, it showed the piece of disc lodged at the L_4-L_5 level and pressing on the L_5 nerve root. A difficult riddle had been translated into a clear indication for a straightforward surgical procedure. I operated to remove the fragment. There was no need to work on the disc, which had already decompressed and healed itself.

Is there any relationship between the CT scan and the new brain-monitoring process known as SEP?

Only in the sense that SEP also aids spinal surgery. SEP (or SSEP) stands for somatosensory evoked potentials. It's an exciting new tool but it is enormously expensive, highly experimental, and still of limited use. SEP is an electrical signal picked up from the cortex of the brain by a series of monitors placed on the patient's head. They measure the way the brain responds to nerve stimulation, usually as it is applied to the limbs.

During some types of spinal surgery, typically during surgery to correct spinal deformity, it is necessary to monitor the functions of the spinal cord. The conventional way of making sure the patient's nervous system is still all right during surgery is to wake him up part way through the operation – not enough to make him fully conscious but enough to get him to respond to commands, such as wiggling his toes.

Now, that practice becomes unnecessary when there is access to a SEP machine. While the spine is manipulated, technicians can monitor the cord's function by stimulating a nerve in the arm or leg and observing a change in the electrical reading from the brain. Any minor alteration in that function will be noted on the instrument, and the surgeon can respond accordingly.

SEP monitoring requires a highly trained team. At the moment, its use is limited to major centers that do a large volume of surgery for spinal deformities, fractures, or tumors. As experience with the equipment grows, however, the machine may well pass from its current experimental phase and become one of the tools of our trade.

Some of the newest work involves measuring the reaction in a single nerve root. SEP can be used in the diagnosis of spinal stenosis to tell exactly which nerve is being squeezed and causing the problem. And it even seems possible to use the equipment during surgery to tell the surgeon just how much bone he must remove to completely decompress the affected root. SEP can't guarantee a good operative result but it certainly can give the doctor a great deal of help along the way.

It sounds like an amazing piece of equipment. Do you see any other use for SEP?

I am excited by its potential for providing a real assessment of pain. We spoke earlier about the difficulty the doctor has in determining the intensity of pain that a patient feels, or in fact whether the patient feels any pain at all. Pain perception is completely subjective, and at the present time we have no way of measuring it. A person may report that he or she has severe pain in an arm or leg, but we have no method of gauging the real strength of that sensation.

Now SEP may provide a means of recording the brain's response to nerve stimulation and therefore to pain. When SEP technology is developed further, we might be able to test and analyze the electrical impulses from a patient's brain to the point where, for the first time, we will actually measure and describe pain objectively.

I read recently about a machine that scans the body by using a magnetic field instead of X-rays. Is this a significant development?

It certainly is. The machine you are referring to performs a technique called magnetic resonance imaging, or MRI. The process is also known as nuclear magnetic resonance or NMR. The MRI equipment operates by subjecting your body to an extremely strong magnet – generating 3,000 to 28,000 times the strength of the earth's magnetic field. This causes the molecules within the body's tissues to align themselves along the magnetic lines of force. You are then bombarded by radio frequency pulses that knock the atomic particles out of alignment. As the nuclei return to their former positions within the magnetic field they give off radio signals of their own. The effect has been likened to lightly tapping a spinning top: it wobbles and then returns to its original upright position. In the nuclei of the atoms, that "wobble" creates a characteristic electrical discharge. A computer records the signals produced specifically by the nuclei of the hydrogen atoms and creates a visual representation of all the hydrogen-containing tissues. Incidentally, hydrogen was selected because so many living tissues contain this element, usually in the form of water, and because no other element responds with a stronger signal than hydrogen does.

Is "visual representation" just Doctor for "picture"?

No, I'm not speaking Doctor here. MRI images are not pictures but finely detailed representations – reconstructions, if you like – of information the computer has gathered and processed. The result is something like the digital recording that is taking over from conventional methods of reproducing sound. As you probably know, when you hear a digital record, you are not hearing a reproduction of the music itself but a numerical reassembly of the notes played by the musicians and recorded on a computer disc. Digital recordings are remarkably "clean" to listen to because they contain no extraneous sounds – only the music that has been translated into numbers and then converted back into sound by the computer.

In an MRI image, you get a visual recreation of what the machine "saw" in the patient's body, but you can understand now why it's incorrect to regard it as an actual picture.

Does an MRI produce a better image than an X-ray or a CT scan?

It's not so much a better image as a different one. X-rays and

CT scans are really shadow-pictures of the body. The image from the MRI computer never existed anywhere else. Compared to an X-ray, the MRI has one big advantage: whereas an X-ray shows only bone and not soft tissue, the MRI shows both and provides much clearer differentiations between them. The difference is less apparent when MRI is compared to a CT scan, but the MRI image is still impressive.

The appearance is certainly different. Because of their low hydrogen content, bones appear black on the MRI, whereas on the X-ray and CT scan they appear white because they block off most of the X-ray beam. The MRI can actually show the difference between a healthy disc and a worn one, by indicating the amount of water they contain. Not only can the MRI show the structure; it can also reveal what it is made of. That's something an X-ray or scan could never do as well. But because the MRI is a representation rather than a direct visual image, it needs a great deal of human interpretation. The surgeon who is used to reading X-rays needs some practice before he can decipher an MRI.

Is that a skill most back doctors have acquired by now?

Not yet. I am enthusiastic about MRI, but the machines are expensive and scarce. The process is just coming into its own for the diagnosis of back problems, but it's bound to have a major impact on the decision-making process in surgical procedures.

Is the high cost of MRI machines responsible for the time lag?

It's one reason; but MRI is still in its early stage of development. At the moment, it can't quite do everything a CT scan can do. For example, from a CT scan I can get a much clearer picture of the vertebrae with slices as thin as 1.5 mm – less than 6/100ths of an inch. The MRI, at the present time, hasn't reached that degree of precision.

Is the patient in any danger from the magnetic field of an MRI?

No one can answer that question with absolute certainty, but by all indications so far, there is no danger. Thousands of patients have had MRI images taken and have been monitored carefully, with no evidence of side effects of any kind. In assessing the risks from the radio frequency impulses, some authorities have estimated that the present strength could be 100 times more powerful before there was any cause for concern.

There are special exceptions, however. Patients who have cardiac pacemakers or metal implants of any kind must avoid MRI. The extreme magnetism would knock the pacemaker out of commission and cause a harmful reaction from any other metallic implant.

So far, MRI machines have presented only one minor drawback for patients: people who are troubled by claustrophobia find it difficult to climb into the MRI chamber and remain there for the necessary twenty to thirty minutes.

I see the MRI as the wave of the future for diagnostic work, partly because it is non-invasive and it completely avoids the concern some patients have about exposure to radiation. The MRI computer can even color the images and produce a stunning display of living anatomy as it has never been seen before.

My doctor was talking about another computerized instrument, a densometer. What is that?

It's not as dramatic as the MRI, but in some ways it's just as exciting. The dual photon densometer promises to revolutionize the diagnosis of osteoporosis. As you will recall, osteoporosis is a condition in which there is a reduction in normal bone mass below the level needed to maintain skeletal support. This is normal with aging, and it is not painful in itself, but it makes the bones susceptible to fracture, which can lead to problems that are both painful and disabling.

Until now, the onset of osteoporosis has often been hard to detect because we have not had an accurate method of measuring bone density. Conventional X-rays are not up to this task. Thirty to 50 percent of the bone mass can disappear before routine X-rays are able to detect any difference.

A more direct method of assessing osteoporosis is the bone biopsy – that is, removing a small sample of bone for laboratory study and analysis. But that's an operation, a painful process that still produces results which can be unreliable, since it is impossible to be sure that the sample taken is typical of the other bones.

Now they have come up with a computerized measuring technique which, even in its early stages of development, is capable of analyzing bone density with amazing precision. A specific radioisotope is injected into the patient's bloodstream. As in a conventional bone scan, the material is taken up by the bones, where it remains for a short while. But unlike the isotope normally used, the new compound emits radiation on two distinct frequencies. A computer records both levels and performs some complex calculations on the two pieces of information. Then it conveniently prints out the percentage of bone loss, comparing it with the average for a person of the same age and sex, and in some cases even estimating the probability of a fracture.

Both dual photon densometry and magnetic resonance imaging are two excellent examples of the new medical tools that will soon enable us to diagnose and treat back problems with unprecedented accuracy and effectiveness.

12. ANYONE FOR SURGERY?

In a medical world seemingly divided between "cutting doctors" and "talking doctors" I feel comfortable in both camps. Although I spend almost half my working days in the operating room, the patients I treat there represent only a small fraction of the backache victims I see. For the others, the appropriate treatments involve less dramatic action – physical therapy, exercise, good posture, and healthy living habits – all constructive ways of working with nature to encourage the healing process.

Because I put so much effort into counseling my patients in back care, many people conclude, quite erroneously, that I disapprove of surgery, or at least that I am reluctant to operate on any back patient except as a last resort.

This isn't true. My low ratio of surgery cases is based on a perfectly sound principle: to be remedied by the scalpel, a back problem must be structural, localized, and specific – an unstable joint or pressure on a nerve root. There is no practical surgical procedure for repairing generalized wear and tear down the length of the spine, and I have yet to acquire forceps capable of reaching into a patient's back and simply plucking out the pain. Even when the trouble is localized to a specific structure, surgery isn't usually the answer.

Most back problems, in other words, are inoperable. Which is not to say that they are hopeless but only that they call for non-surgical treatment. An operation is not a last resort but a particular remedy suitable for selected cases. Whenever these cases are referred to me, I recommend surgery with an alacrity that would surprise those who consider me an "anti-surgery surgeon."

On the other hand, I flatly refuse to operate when I'm convinced surgery is the wrong way to solve the problem and is unlikely to succeed. Not long ago, a woman walked into my office and announced: "I need a back operation." After reading my first book, she had diagnosed herself as the victim of Type Three back trouble (a pinched nerve) and had decided surgery was the remedy. When I examined her I found she was wrong on both counts. I explained this to her, declined to operate – and lost her as a patient. I have no doubt she has since been making the rounds in search of a "cutting doctor" who will do as she asks.

In contrast, I remember a genuine Type Three patient who should have had surgery. The man had been lifting some files out of the back seat of his car when he lost his balance and twisted his body. Three months later, he came to me, and the CT scan I ordered showed he had a large disc herniation in his low back. The affected disc was pressing on a nerve root, causing severe pain and a progressive weakness of muscles in one buttock and the calf of one leg. I recommended surgery and predicted that he had a 90 percent chance of making a complete recovery. Naturally I also discussed the possible complications of the operation, such as infection or local nerve injury, and I stressed the need for continuing back care when the post-operative period was over.

Unfortunately, my warnings must have scared him off. He declined the operation and has been suffering ever since – from inactivity, unemployment, financial problems, his weak leg, and the back pain itself. The choice was his, of course, but clearly he would have been far better off having the operation.

I would feel much happier about both those patients if I had managed to provide them with a clearer perspective of spinal surgery, to help them make better-informed decisions. I hope this chapter will provide that perspective for many back patients facing comparable situations.

Just the idea of having a back operation frightens me. Do many of your patients feel the same way?

Many are frightened by the very word "surgery" and everything they associate with it – from the intimidating atmosphere of the operating room to the possibility of never regaining consciousness after a general anesthetic. Some of them believe the spine is such a complex and mysterious part of the body that the very prospect of having it invaded or disturbed is terrifying.

And that's with *elective* surgery. Imagine an accident victim who is lying in Emergency when a surgeon – a total stranger – walks in and says, "How do you do. I am going to operate on you in about an hour." No wonder patients are frightened. Not just at the thought of surgery but because someone they have never even seen before has just announced he is going to do something drastic to them. Feeling that absolute loss of control, and the need to depend so completely on someone they don't know, must be terrible. In that situation I always take a little extra time to get acquainted with the patient and the family and explain what the surgery is all about.

On the other hand, I have patients who are so convinced they need surgery that they won't follow my advice about doing anything else to help themselves. They just keep waiting for me to agree to operate on them and assume full responsibility for their recovery. They view the operation as an easy way out, often expecting it to alleviate not only their back problem but many of their non-medical complaints as well. Some patients seem to believe back surgery will improve everything from their short temper to their falling hair.

It must be important to know what your surgeon plans to do and how he believes it will help.

Certainly the more you know the more comfortable you will feel. Listen carefully to what you're told, first by your family doctor, and then by the surgeon, who has a responsibility to help you understand your operation. With my patients I spend a lot of time explaining what I'm going to do. I know they have certain expectations, and I know the operation is capable of correcting certain things. It's in everyone's best interest to make sure those two elements match up. If your expectations are unrealistic, you are not likely to be satisfied with the results.

Often, it's a simple matter of clear communication. Although the onus lies primarily on the surgeon, for your own sake as a patient you should do everything you can to make sure the message you're hearing is the message that's intended. If the surgeon says, "You'll be fine in a week," and fails to elaborate, the two of you may have wildly different notions of what that means. You may think being "fine" means suddenly becoming twenty years younger and able to leap tall buildings in a single bound, while he probably means you'll be well enough to get out of hospital, perhaps with a little help.

The only way to overcome such gaps in understanding is to talk. Ask questions. Get an explanation of any point you're unsure about. Clear up any discrepancies between the things you have heard elsewhere and the things your doctor is telling you. You're a rare patient indeed if you don't have at least one or two misconceptions about back surgery. No matter how hard I try to present my patients with a clear picture of the procedure, I'm sure some of them remain convinced, for instance, that I plan to completely remove one or two discs from their spines. That operation, commonly referred to as a "disc removal," actually entails something far less drastic; only the *nucleus* of the disc is removed – and only a part of the nucleus at that.

What *is* back surgery all about? There must be many different kinds of operations or procedures.

Surprisingly there are just two basic types of surgery for common backache, although, as you might suppose, wide variations are practiced within each type.

One is decompression, involving the removal of pressure being exerted on the nerves within the spine. That pressure can come from several sources – a disc bulging into the spinal canal and pressing against a single nerve root or against the dural sac containing the *cauda equina* or, higher up, the spinal cord; a bit of nucleus that has escaped from a disc and lodged somewhere in the canal; a bony growth from a facet joint or the wall of the canal that is reducing the size of the tunnel. If you remember what we said earlier about the four types of backache, you will realize that all the conditions I just mentioned are forms of Type

Three pain (the pinched nerve) or Type Four pain (spinal stenosis). Decompression, broadly speaking, involves removal of whatever is pressing on the nerve.

The other basic operation is stabilization, or fusion, as it is commonly called, which is a remedy for Type One and Type Two pain. It involves fusing two or more vertebrae together to eliminate any painful movement. The problem may be either worn facet joints rubbing together, or a bulging disc that is no longer serving as the firm cushion it was intended to be. To join two vertebrae, the surgeon bridges the joints and disc space between them with pieces of bone that are permanently incorporated into both vertebrae. The joints are immobilized, the disc is replaced by solid bone, and the two vertebrae become fused into one structure.

Do some back patients need both types of operations – decompression *and* fusion?

Yes, in some patients with Type Three or Type Four pain, decompression may be combined with fusion. For instance, after a decompression that clears up the problem of a pinched nerve, the surgeon might find that removing the required amount of material has produced a mechanical instability requiring a fusion.

Are the two types of operation performed at the same time?

Sometimes. If a stenosis patient needed several facet joints removed for decompression, the surgeon could anticipate a degree of instability that would need stabilizing, and he might very well perform both procedures during the one session.

Are most back operations successful?

If by successful you mean that the operation gets rid of your symptoms, the answer is yes, they are. Your pain is gone and you can function normally. Realistically, you can't expect surgery to transform a worn old back into a brand new one; that kind of success will always elude us.

Success depends on two important conditions. First, the operation must be done for the right reason: you must have a condition that can be remedied by the proposed surgical procedure. And second, the operation must be done properly. If these basic conditions are met, the chances of success are excellent. As you might expect, however, the prospects are better for some types of back surgery than for others.

The back operation with the best success rate is one of the decompression operations, the simple discotomy. In this procedure, the surgeon cuts out a small portion of the bony plate on the back of the vertebrae (the plate is called the *lamina* and this part of the operation is called a laminectomy). Through that little hole into the spinal canal the surgeon can reach the disc and remove the bulge that is pressing on the nerve. Nine out of ten patients who undergo a routine laminectomy and discotomy get rid of their symptoms and return to normal living. The success rate for the simple discotomy is high because it is a straightforward operation for which the indications are very clear.

For the benefit of those who like to pick up a little Doctor language now and then, I should explain that the suffix "otomy" means "to put a hole in," and so the first part of the operation really ought to be called a laminotomy. The suffix "ectomy" means "to remove," and so the second phase of the operation should actually be called a "partial discectomy." But in common surgical jargon these "pure" terms have been slightly corrupted, and the procedure is known instead as a "laminectomy-discotomy."

Do all the people who need simple discotomies have the same problems?

Yes, with minor variations. The symptoms include a predominance of leg pain and other leg complaints, such as loss of power in certain muscle groups, decreased sensation, or the disappearance of a reflex. The exact pattern depends on the specific nerve root involved and that depends on the precise location of the disc rupture. The patient's complaints either fail to get better with well-controlled bed rest and physical therapy, or they actually grow worse. When the indications are that clear, surgery is likely to be done at the right time, and the chances of success are consequently very good.

Other forms of decompression surgery may be carried out for problems that are hard to determine so precisely, such as an area of spinal stenosis causing *cauda equina* claudication, and accordingly their success rate is somewhat lower. Even at that, surgical enlargement of a short length of the spinal canal to reduce nerve pressure has a success rate well over 85 percent.

The reason for that lack of precision isn't hard to understand. The surgeon may correctly diagnose the problem as one involving pressure from bony overgrowth in the canal without being able to tell exactly how much bone needs to come out. Consequently he may go in and remove some bone without taking quite as much as he should, thus failing to relieve all the pressure on the nerve. Or the surgeon may err in the opposite direction, overdoing the bone removal. Destroying too much of the roof and sides of the tunnel can allow an excessive growth of scar tissue, which can choke the nerve as much as the original stenosis did. And eliminating the entire posterior joint structure will lead to segmental instability.

Instability caused by decompression surgery is not nearly so common today as it was in the sixties, when we knew less than we know now about spinal stenosis and its remedies. In those days it was not unusual for surgeons to remove the posterior elements of four or five vertebrae. Although the early results were satisfactory, over half the patients had their back problems return within two years. Some had spines that were so unstable that the vertebrae actually began to move out of alignment. The only remedy was fusion, which was a pretty "iffy" proposition with so many levels of the spine involved.

What about the success rate for fusion operations generally?

If you have a condition where you need a fusion at just one level – that is, where only two vertebrae are to be joined into a single unit – the chances of success are good, approaching 90 percent. The percentage is slightly lower for a fusion at two levels, and lower still for three levels, which is pretty well the surgical limit in cases of ordinary Type One or Type Two back pain.

Instability is a subtle and complicated condition that's hard to assess. Although one level of your spine might show definite signs of wear with abnormal movement, the neighboring levels may also be involved to a lesser but significant degree. By stabilizing that one level, I will be shifting the load to the other levels, which may consequently become unstable. Because of these inherent uncertainties, I never recommend or perform a fusion unless I am convinced that the person is seriously disabled, with pain that cannot be controlled by a rigorous exercise and training program. And when I make the decision to operate, I have to take into account the fact that fusion will set up new conditions that can cause new trouble.

Fusion is generally a larger operation than decompression. Because more muscle is stripped away from the bone to gain access, it causes more scar tissue to form. Scar tissue is tender stuff and can cause considerable local discomfort for a year or more. Usually the bone used in the fusion is obtained from the patient's pelvis, and this "donor site" becomes a second source of pain during the convalescence.

All in all, it's a process so complicated that no one can say with certainty that a fusion operation will get rid of all the pain, even if the bones unite to provide a solid bridge between the adjacent vertebrae.

To make matters a little more confusing, a few patients will have good results from their fusions with excellent pain relief and return of function, while their X-rays clearly show the operation has failed to produce a bony connection between the vertebrae. In other words, although the surgery was a technical failure it was a clinical success.

Perhaps the one exception to the uncertainty about low-back fusions is the operation for spondylolithesis at L_5. This is a condition where a defect in the normally solid bridge between the upper and lower joints of the last mobile vertebra allows the body of the bone to slip forward. Fusing to restore normal stability is one case where a technically successful operation almost always solves the problem.

You must walk a tightrope, trying to help a patient understand what the chances and risks are, and yet not discourage or frighten off the person who would probably benefit greatly from surgery.

That's exactly right. Like most other surgeons, I try to achieve what has become known as "informed consent." That means asking the patient to accept treatment with a full understanding of both the positive and negative results that could ensue.

Is this idea of "informed consent" a new concept for surgeons?

Yes – in the deliberate and expanded manner that is customary today. The traditional routine of signing the consent form merely gave your permission, whether you understood or not. The evolution of informed consent as a concept was pointed up to me recently by a friend who described an experience he had about thirty-five years ago. As a young man, my friend needed minor surgery for the removal of a couple of sebaceous cysts in his scalp. A few days before the operation, the surgeon told him that while the operation was pretty routine, there was always the chance that the cysts would not come out completely; some portion might remain to cause trouble in the future. When my friend mentioned this caution to his uncle, a retired doctor, the uncle laughed and said: "He's just making up excuses in advance, in case he botches the operation."

The uncle's response shows how most doctors viewed such cautions in earlier times. Today, with the public more aware of surgical risks and with doctors feeling more vulnerable to malpractice suits, the surgeon, for ethical and legal reasons, must forewarn the patient by spelling out the potential risks entailed in any procedure. If he fails to do that, he could be accused of operating without the patient's informed consent.

I fully approve of informed consent. As you suggested, however, it's sometimes a hard principle to apply. Where do I draw the line between informing my patient as fully as necessary and scaring him out of his wits? It's easy to describe what I think I am going to achieve and how well I hope it will go. It's much more difficult to dwell on all the possible causes of failure and still maintain the patient's confidence in my ability as a surgeon.

And my approach won't be the same for all my patients. Each of them is a unique individual with his or her own intelligence, emotional makeup, and expectations based on a mixture of real experience, valid information, vivid imagination, and folklore.

For most operations, we know the percentages of successes and failures, but these don't really tell the whole story. As a patient, you are a person, not a statistic. There is not much consolation in having known beforehand that the general success rate is 90 percent if it turns out that the success of your own surgery is zero. So I attempt to explain where the problems may come from and what can be done about them should they arise. Most of all I want the patient to realize why in his or her particular case the operation is worth the potential risks.

This concept of informed consent is something to keep in mind, against the day when you may have to listen to the pros and cons involved in having your own back surgery. If your doctor seems to be telling you more than you want to hear about the risks, remember: if you are to share in the decision intelligently, you must have a thorough understanding of what you're getting into.

If I have an operation on my back, is it possible I will need surgery later on for the same problem?

The majority of people who have one operation never have or need to have a second one. If the results of your surgery have been good for at least a year after the recovery period, you can be reasonably sure that it was a technical success and you won't need an encore, at least not for the same problem. On the other hand, if your original trouble returns within six months, a second operation to try to make things better usually fails. Unless a new problem can be demonstrated clearly, more surgery is not often the answer.

I have been presented with all too many sad examples of second surgery. On one occasion I was asked to provide a consultation on another surgeon's patient who had serious problems. The woman (I'll call her Mrs. Wallace) had been through three back operations, all of them fusions. All three operations had failed, and she still had disabling back pain.

Mrs. Wallace had just had another myelogram, and I could see that while the attempts at fusion had partially stabilized several of the worn areas, her spine was a long way from normal. At every level of her low back there was one problem or another – here some narrowing of the spinal canal, there a bulging disc, here an arthritic joint, somewhere else a failed fusion. Through a combination of normal aging, natural wear and tear, and three operations, the poor woman had a spine that was beyond salvaging.

And, as I suspected, I had been invited there with more than simple consultation in mind. Mrs. Wallace wanted me to operate on her. She had read my first book and made up her mind that my surgical skill was the answer to her problem. I know she was disappointed when I said there was no operation I could perform that would help her. But it was true. There was not even anything new to be found that would justify any drastic change in her treatment. Every problem I spotted in her myelogram was already known to her own surgeon, who had performed those three failed operations. I offered her a program of chronic pain management and exercise, but Mrs. Wallace clearly wasn't interested. I left the case with the distinct impression that her surgeon would soon give in and take her into surgery for a fourth round. I wish them both well but I don't give them much chance of success.

I gather you don't hold much hope for a third or fourth spinal operation.

That's putting it mildly. I often say to patients, "Your first chance is your best chance, and your second chance is your last chance." Unless, as rarely happens, the back surgery is for a completely different condition.

I first made that observation many years ago, and it was borne out later by a study done in co-operation with the Ontario Workers' Compensation Board. We reviewed cases where patients had undergone two or more unsuccessful back operations, looking for reasons why the surgery failed. We found that the most common reason for the failure of a second operation was the same as the reason for the failure of the first: most of these patients shouldn't have had surgery at all. Typically, the indications for the original surgery were unconvincing or confused. The patients had few if any clinical findings that suggested the need for any operation. Some patients had normal myelograms; others had myelograms that did not match up with their clinical findings. Almost all the other tests that were done revealed nothing significant.

It was hardly surprising, then, that those first operations had less than six months of apparent success, followed by a recurrence of the same old trouble. Having undergone the original surgery for inappropriate reasons, these people went through the same process all over again, with the same poor result.

Of course there were other cases, too, where surgery failed the first time around, even though it had been the proper course to follow.

Why would surgery fail if it was done for the right reason?

Perhaps it wasn't performed properly or thoroughly enough, or maybe the patient didn't follow the doctor's instructions about post-operative care. Or there could have been a complication or a second problem that wasn't diagnosed at the outset.

However, in cases where the need for surgery was clear from the beginning, the second round of surgery undertaken to salvage those first-time failures had a high rate of success. When it came to a third operation, no matter how valid the indications had been for the first two, the chances of improvement fell dramatically. Which is why I say that when it comes to back surgery, your second chance is your last chance.

Are you saying, then, that it's futile for anyone to have more than two back operations?

Generally speaking, yes, it is, particularly if the successive operations are all intended to remedy the same disorder. It's a different matter if new back problems develop after successful surgery. One patient of mine has gone through three operations for herniated discs – twice at the same level and the third at the level below. The operations took place a year apart, each time near Christmas. The timing and regularity of her surgery became a bit of an unhappy joke between us. But every operation was justified and all of them succeeded. In each instance she had fully recovered and remained symptom-free for longer than six months, the critical period for gauging the potential success for "second try" surgery. She simply had the rare misfortune of developing three separate disc herniations (one at the site of previous surgery) on three separate occasions.

That patient was lucky: her last surgery, many Christmases ago, left her with a functional, pain-free back. Another patient of mine wasn't as fortunate. He had had a series of operations, each of which solved an immediate problem but left his spine less stable. His original problem was a routine case of stenosis; several nerves were being squeezed in an abnormally narrow part of the spinal canal. I corrected that problem with a decompression operation. Three years later the man was struck by a car, injuring his spine. Our findings indicated the need for another decompression, and when I operated I found a distinct ridge of scar tissue right across the area we had opened up earlier. The impact of the accident had either added more scar or disrupted a comfortable balance between the scar left from my first surgery and the local nerve roots. I removed the excessive fibrous tissue, enlarged the canal a little more, and my patient got better.

Then, a full year later, his back pain recurred, and I decided he needed a third decompression. This time he had developed a large ingrowth of scar at the upper end of the previous decompression. Scarring, as you probably know, is one of the body's natural responses to injury, including surgery. It produces many benefits but it has its drawbacks; scar tissue can choke off a nerve and cause severe pain. In this man's case, I felt there was little choice but to remove that ingrowth of scar along with some more of the bone on the back of his spine and hope for the best. Unfortunately, that additional bone loss deprived his spine of still more of its natural stability. The only possible remedy for his fourth recurrence of disabling back pain was yet another round of surgery – this time a fusion, which, I am happy to say, was the last operation the man needed. He still has chronic back pain, but he can control it well enough to lead a normal life.

It's worth noting that while every one of those operations was a success in itself, the earlier surgery made the subsequent operations necessary. While it's true that the final outcome in this case was satisfactory, it was far from perfect. If you are facing the prospect of surgery, don't limit your discussion with the doctor to the immediate problem. Consider the long-term effects of the operation on the function of your spine, the chance of increased trouble in other areas of your back, or even the chance of a recurrence of the original difficulty. Be sure you understand your role in the rehabilitation process and whether there will be any need for a permanent adjustment of your activities.

What about neck surgery? How is it different from operations on the lower back?

There are a few significant differences. The canal in the cervical spine contains the spinal cord rather than the separate nerve roots found in the low back. The cord is very sensitive to pressure, and for this reason the operations are designed to avoid any pulling or pushing on it. And, of course, damage to the spinal cord would have far more serious consequences than injury to a single nerve root lower down.

But the indications and techniques of surgery are otherwise much the same. The most common reasons for an operation are: painful wear in a disc (Type Two); or pressure on a nerve root as it leaves the spine (Type Three). This pressure produces pain or loss of function in the arm or hand. Most neck problems can be managed with non-surgical treatment, however, and of all the patients I see with neck pain, only about 1 percent require an operation.

Decompression operations can be done through the back of the neck in the same way we perform decompressions in the lumbar spine. But because of concerns about moving the spinal cord aside to reach the disc, many surgeons make their approach from the front. A small incision is made on one side of the neck and then deepened through the muscles before passing between the carotid artery (a major artery to the brain) on one side and the trachea (the windpipe) on the other.

The front of the spine can be seen at the bottom of the wound, and most of the nucleus of the troublesome disc is easily removed through a hole cut in its outer shell. It is possible to work all the way to the back of the disc to eliminate bulges pressing on the nerves in the spinal canal.

Because the neck is more flexible than the low back and because the frontal approach removes a large amount of the nucleus of the disc, this technique usually produces a degree of instability. For that reason, decompression is almost always combined with a fusion. A small block of bone taken from the pelvis is fitted into the disc space between the vertebral bodies.

In other cases, such as when treating a major injury to the facet joints of the neck, a fusion can be done from behind, in much the same way as we usually fuse the low back.

After surgery the patient wears a rigid collar but is usually able to be up within a day or two. Until the bone graft forms a solid union, which takes about three months, the neck must be protected. During convalescence, the donor site on the pelvis often hurts more than the fusion in the neck.

Are neck operations generally safe and successful?

Yes. Although most people don't need an operation to solve their neck problems, when surgery is required the success rate is high. The same complications that sometimes result from low-back surgery can occur after neck surgery, but they rarely do. Special care is taken in handling the major vessels to the head, in protecting the spinal cord, and in making sure nothing is done to disturb the nerves that control the vocal cords.

What circumstances would prompt you to recommend back surgery for me?

Since the symptoms and the treatment wouldn't be the same for every type of back problem, I'll describe my approach to a typical situation involving the commonest form of back surgery, the discotomy (which really ought to be called a partial discectomy, since only some of the center, or nucleus, of the disc is removed).

By the time we considered a discotomy, you would probably have seen me several times, for pain that is in your back but much worse in your lower leg and foot. Under my direction, you would have gone through several weeks of conservative management consisting primarily of bed rest and gentle extension exercises.

My decision to consider an operation would be prompted by your signs and symptoms either failing to improve or growing worse. And that raises a very important point: I would not suggest an operation simply because you have pain. I would have to be convinced you are suffering from a loss of nerve function that could not be restored through rest and non-surgical treatment.

How could you tell if there is a loss of normal function in a nerve?

Earlier, when we discussed the causes of common backache, we talked about the tests for irritation of a nerve root. We also discussed the ways to tell whether a certain nerve is failing to conduct impulses properly. These examinations would help me make my decision.

Nerve irritation, the source of most of your leg pain, can be measured by the straight-leg-raising test. I'd have you lie flat on your back with your knee extended while I raised your leg. If you felt pain in the back of your thigh, calf, or foot with an elevation of less than sixty degrees, I would know you had nerve irritation. Other tests could indicate the same problem. For instance, if pressure applied behind your knee caused pain to spread up or down your leg, there would be abnormal irritation somewhere in the sciatic nerve.

If you had a loss of sensation in a specific area of the leg, an absent reflex at the knee or ankle, or, most important of all, decreased power in certain groups of muscles, I would know that one of the nerves coming from the lumbar spine was unable to carry its normal signals. The failure of these functions and their lack of recovery over a period of time are factors in determining the need for surgery.

Even at this point, however, I might bring you into hospital for several days to see whether complete bed rest would improve your condition. At home there are just too many temptations to get up and join the family for dinner or help with the chores. Once you were in that hospital bed you'd stay there. You could get up to use the toilet or take a daily shower, but that's all. Otherwise, you'd be lying down, even while eating your meals or watching TV. The physical therapists would keep a close eye on your resting positions and direct a program of gentle exercise. No sitting back against plumped-up pillows all day. As I said earlier, sitting is hard on your back, and in this situation it could defeat the purpose of your time in hospital.

You'd be surprised at how many of my patients begin to get well during that short stay. Often, those few days of bed rest under close supervision are enough to start them on the road to recovery. They can go home without surgery, get some more rest, and then start on a long-term program to get their backs in shape.

What would happen if I didn't respond well to hospital rest? Would you automatically schedule me for the discotomy?

Not automatically. The next items on your agenda would be a few diagnostic tests. Special studies would be carried out, along with some ordinary X-rays of your low back, routine blood work, and a general physical assessment. You might be given a myelogram or a CT scan or both, to determine the exact location of your bulging disc. If the results of your tests confirmed my diagnosis and located the problem, you would be scheduled for surgery.

What do you do, exactly, when you perform the discotomy?

It's a straightforward matter of going in and removing the nucleus of the disc that's bulging out against the nerve.

I begin by making a one- to two-inch-long incision in your back, at the appropriate spot, as determined by your myelogram or CT scan. On the way to my destination, I carefully strip away the muscles that block my entry and temporarily retract them to one side. Next, I remove a small portion of the roof of the spinal canal (a section of the bony plate, or *lamina*, and the yellow ligament, or *ligamentum flavum*, that spans the space between the bones).

Once inside the canal I gently push the nerve sac and root aside to reach the disc located on the floor of the tunnel. The bulge is usually quite easy to see; the inflammation makes it look like a large pimple. Curled up in the middle of that bump is the material that escaped from the center of the disc. After extracting the loose fragment I may or may not attempt to clean out the remainder of the nucleus still contained within the disc's outer shell. I know it's impossible to remove all of it, but I can probably take out about 75 percent. I don't remove the thick walls that bind the disc to the vertebrae on either side. Nor do I worry about the hollow that I've left in the center of the disc, since this will fill harmlessly with scar tissue stronger and more resilient than the part of the nucleus I removed.

Whether or not I proceed to remove those portions of the nucleus remaining within the disc will depend on how I judge the situation. Usually the surgeon scrapes out all the nucleus he can get, to ensure that another loose piece isn't lurking inside the disc waiting to cause more trouble. But if I find that the *anulus* – the outer shell of the disc – has healed so well that no more nucleus can get out, I'd be foolish to disturb what nature has already mended.

Once I have removed the necessary amount of material, it's just a matter of withdrawing from the site, covering the exposed dura (nerve sac) with a thin layer of fat to reduce future scarring, moving back the muscles that were pushed aside, and closing up the incision. The whole operation is briefer than the average movie – sixty to ninety minutes – and a lot less bloody than some.

How am I likely to feel right after a discotomy? Will my old pain be gone?

Yes. The first thing you are likely to notice when you wake up is that your leg pain has disappeared, although the incision in your back will be sore. You will be told that if you need to get up in the night to use the toilet, you are free to do so, and you will be encouraged to start walking the next day as much as you can. You won't even need a corset.

On the second day, your leg will still be pain free, but you will begin to realize your back is hurting more and more. I always warn my patients about this in advance. I tell them what other patients have told me: after a discotomy you feel as though you've been kicked by a horse in the small of the back. The pain is the result of muscle bruising, which occurred when I pushed those muscles aside to get at the disc. Muscles don't like being pushed around. They gradually become swollen and sore, and they complain accordingly.

Your back pain, however, will be quite different from the pain you had before your operation. The new pain will be easier to endure, like a tender bruise that's sensitive to the touch. Something about the quality of the pain makes most patients realize that it is temporary and will be gone in a few days. I remember one patient who had his discotomy on Friday morning and was out enjoying dinner in a restaurant on Sunday afternoon.

Even during those uncomfortable first days, you can be up and around, although you'll be moving cautiously. You'll learn to roll onto one side and then push yourself up to a sitting position to avoid stressing the area of your surgery. Walking is good because it stimulates the circulation in your legs, and that helps prevent blood clots from forming in the veins there. It keeps your lungs working well. And it's a morale booster. You'll find yourself thinking, "Hey – I'm getting better already!" The current emphasis on early activity is quite a change from the old days when patients were kept in bed for a week or more after simple disc surgery.

For the first week or two you can do anything you want, but you should avoid sitting for extended periods, since that puts quite a load on the area of the surgery. You are encouraged to stand, lie down, or perch somewhere, leaning with your backside against a counter or window-ledge.

How long will I have to stay in the hospital?

After simple disc surgery, you can usually expect to go home in less than three or four days. Some surgeons keep their patients in hospital for a week; others pride themselves on sending people home after forty-eight hours or less. The general trend these days is to get patients up and out as quickly as possible.

What are the chances of a complication following a discotomy?

The risks are small. But there are potential complications from the anesthetic, the chance of damaging a nerve root during surgery, and the possibility of a wound infection later on. You must also be aware that for a few vulnerable patients, typically those well along in years or with previous medical problems, the stress of an operation and the period of convalescence which follows can precipitate a heart attack or a stroke, or a blood clot in the lungs. I often remind my patients that having back surgery is not like having a haircut; there are a number of potentially serious complications. I hasten to add that the chance of trouble is small, less than two in a hundred for all complications combined. And the surgical team is highly skilled in avoiding or minimizing these problems.

One minor complication that can cause you a good deal of pain is an attack of muscle spasms in your back. I'm not referring to the bit of backache that results from bruising the muscles during surgery; I'm talking about really bad muscle cramps quite unlike anything you felt before the operation. If these occur, they will likely start soon after surgery, while you are still in hospital.

How long do spasms like that usually last?

That's unpredictable. They might last just a few days, or they could drag on for several weeks. The only consolation is that they eventually end. I have never seen any, or heard of any, that didn't.

What can be done to stop the muscles from cramping?

Unfortunately, not much. Unlike other kinds of spasms, which may respond to even a single treatment of massage, manipulation, heat, or medication, these post-operative cramps seldom yield readily. The important thing is to avoid panic, which will only make them worse.

From all I have just said you may be vowing never to undergo a discotomy no matter what your doctor advises. But you must not lose sight of the fact that the removal of a disc fragment is an excellent decompression procedure with an extremely high rate of success and an extremely low risk of complication.

Would my chance of success be better if I had a microdiscotomy?

Microdiscotomy means that the surgeon uses an operating microscope while performing the surgery. The actual operation is much the same as the one I just described. Increased magnification may make it easier to avoid damage to a nerve root, but for a competent surgeon this is not necessarily a difficult feat even without a microscope. Microdiscotomy also means the use of specially designed surgical instruments, smaller and more delicate than those normally employed. And viewing the wound through the microscope may make the surgeon more aware of minor problems and the need to maintain a meticulous operative technique.

But the microscope has its disadvantages as well. The apparatus is large, awkward, and very expensive. Positioning it above the operative field is time-consuming and may contaminate the sterile area. So the operation usually takes longer, and there have been cases where significant pathology was missed because it lay outside the surgeon's necessarily restricted field of view.

The indications are the same no matter which style of discotomy is selected, as are the chances of success or complications. I have no objection to microdiscotomy so long as it isn't regarded as a guaranteed method or used as a gimmick to attract business and raise the cost of surgery.

What about other kinds of decompression operations?

The discotomy is the commonest type. As I mentioned earlier, getting to the disc usually means removing a portion of the *lamina*, the bone that forms part of the roof of the spinal canal. Occasionally, removal of this bone alone is done to eliminate nerve pressure, and the procedure is labeled a decompressive laminectomy. As far as the patient's perception goes, there is virtually no difference between a discotomy and a laminectomy.

Another fairly common but slightly different form of decompression is the type performed for spinal stenosis – removal of bony growths that are narrowing the spinal canal and interfering with nerve function. This is usually a more difficult operation than a simple discotomy, because it's harder to remove bone than it is to remove loose fragments of disc. For this reason, the operation takes longer and often means pushing aside more muscle, since the bone removal may be required from both sides of the tunnel. In addition to the decompressive laminectomy, the surgery may entail partial removal of the walls of the canal and the overhanging facet joints. Compared to the discotomy, decompression for stenosis leaves a lot more scar tissue and requires a longer period for full recovery.

During recovery, you may need to wear some sort of back brace or support, which is unnecessary after a simple discotomy; otherwise, the post-op situation is much the same. Often, you will wake up with your pre-operative back pain and your leg symptoms gone, although you won't know that for sure until you are up and around again.

Can you judge beforehand whether decompression is needed on one or both sides?

Yes, I'm usually able to tell from the CT scan and my assessment of your signs and symptoms. Once in a while, there is a disparity between what I see on the X-rays and the clinical examination. My physical findings may suggest that significant compression exists only on one side, while the CT scan shows bilateral narrowing. In that situation there may be a case to be made for decompressing both sides: the potential trouble is real enough to justify preventive surgery. I generally adhere to the old adage, "If it ain't broke, don't fix it," but I don't allow it to overrule my judgment in a specific situation.

I gather that, compared to a discotomy, decompression for stenosis is a more difficult operation for the patient to get through.

That's true. The stenotic patient doesn't always get the immediate relief felt by the discotomy patient. If you have extensive surgery for stenosis you will probably be required to stay in bed a little longer afterwards, and you'll likely take two or three months to get back to your normal routine instead of the few weeks needed by most discotomy patients. But even though your progress may be a little slower, you will likely enjoy some early improvement, and within the first few days, your doctor should be able to predict a good outcome for you.

What complications may follow decompression for stenosis?

The complications, if any, are about the same as for a discotomy. If the decompression has required a great deal of bone removal, there may also be problems with instability. It's possible to remove so much of the posterior part of the spine that the joints begin to slip out of place. That doesn't commonly occur, but it can happen, and if it does, you may need stabilization. Because of this potential problem, surgeons sometimes decide to perform a fusion during the same operation.

Now, tell me about fusion. Is there a single, standard procedure for it, or are there several different types?

Spinal fusion can take many forms. Basically, any time you join one vertebra to another with a bridge of bone, that's a spinal fusion. You can fuse one level, two levels, or multiple levels. Multiple-level fusions are not usually practical for common backache, but they are used to correct a deformity such as the abnormal, side-to-side curvature found in scoliosis patients. When it is severe, the curvature can be partially straightened and then held in the corrected position with a fusion.

It's possible to fuse segments of the spine using only bone (routinely taken from the patient's pelvis). To fuse several adjacent levels of the spine into one unit, we often secure the vertebrae with plates, rods, or wires to prevent movement while the bone graft heals. You can fuse from the back, from the front, or from the sides of the spinal column. As you can imagine, each of these techniques and approaches has its advantages, and each poses its own set of problems.

What are the usual reasons for fusing in cases of common backache?

The reason is always instability, which in most cases will have developed as a result of normal wear and tear in the discs and facet joints. The worn or damaged areas are believed to produce pain when they move, and since fusion stops movement it should eliminate the pain. Occasionally, the spine may become unstable as a result of previous remedial surgery, and a fusion will be needed to maintain normal alignment.

Please describe a typical fusion.

The routine fusion is done without metal, usually involves just one or two levels, and is approached from the back. The surgery takes more time than a simple disc removal. It usually lasts from one and a half to three hours.

To perform the operation, I make an incision about three inches long at the appropriate location. By pushing aside muscles, ligaments, and fat, much as I do for a discotomy, I arrive at the vertebrae which are to be fused together. I enlarge the exposure so that I can see not only the *laminae* but the full extent of the facet joints and outsides of the vertebrae down to the transverse processes, those little bony "wings" that serve as muscle attachments. Now I use a chisel-like instrument to rough up the surface of the bones and destroy the slippery linings within the joints where the grafting is to take place. This deliberate damage causes the body to activate its healing processes, without which the fusion could not take place.

With the fusion site open and ready, I make a second incision, this time along the back of your pelvis. When I get down to the bone, I slice off several strips of the outer bone to reveal the spongy bone inside. I use a gouge to remove this spongy bone in the form of thick little ribbons.

Next I return to the first incision and pack those little ribbons and strips into the facet joints and onto the damaged surfaces I prepared along each side of the vertebrae. These pieces bridge the adjacent segments. As the body reacts to this situation, it treats that bone graft as fragments that have broken away from the spine. With normal healing the graft is gradually incorporated until the new bone and the two vertebrae are fused into a single, solid unit.

That, essentially, is what fusion surgery is all about, although variations are always being introduced in efforts to improve the results. For instance, I often approach the spine through two incisions on either side of the mid-line, splitting the spinal muscles rather than pushing them aside. This gives me a better view of the bed where I want to lay my graft.

An aunt of mine had a fusion operation some years ago and had to spend several weeks on a special bed – some kind of rotating frame. Is that standard post-operative treatment?

Not any longer. There was a time when fusion patients routinely remained for several weeks on a turning frame so that they could be rolled over without any movement of the back until healing of the fusion was well along. Such treatment, however, is generally passé now, thanks to improvements in our surgical techniques.

What improvements in surgical techniques have made the turning frame unnecessary?

In the earlier techniques, strips of bone graft were placed behind the vertebrae directly on the *laminae* or wired to the large posterior projections located under the surface of the skin. In that position, the grafts were quite vulnerable; even a slight amount of movement could prevent them from adhering to the spine.

In the newer techniques, we locate the fusion towards the front of the vertebrae near the point known as the axis of rotation. To understand the principle involved, think of the last time you rode on a merry-go-round. You probably noticed that the closer you were positioned to the outer edge, the faster the ride and the more ground you covered. If you wanted to reduce the amount of movement, you picked a horse near the middle. Similarly, in the newer types of fusion we place the graft as close as possible to the center of rotation, where movement is minimal. Since there is less danger of disturbing the fusion, the patient doesn't need to remain immobile on a turning frame.

The more extensive fusions undertaken to correct major structural damage or significant deformities such as scoliosis now routinely use some form of internal fixation. Excellent techniques have been developed to insert screws through the walls of the spinal canal into the large vertebral body in front. Those screws can be used to secure plates, rods, or heavy cables. In other methods, the devices are held in place by wires that loop around the bones in the roof of the canal. To correct a scoliotic curve, the surgeon may use hooks that slip under the *laminae* and are pushed apart or pulled together along thick metal rods. But no matter what implant is selected, its primary purpose is to provide temporary stability while the bone graft slowly converts the multiple mobile segments into a single, rigid piece of bone.

Even after a multiple-level fusion with solid internal fixation, the patient is often able to get up within a week, wearing a carefully fitted brace. A body cast can be made and then used to mold a plastic shell to cover the entire back. The patient will wear this shell day and night for months until the fusion is solid.

With all these advances, it has become unnecessary for a patient with a spinal fusion to use the turning frame or even to undergo prolonged bed rest. Such progress has also opened the way for surgical treatment of previously unsolved spinal disorders.

I've heard that some hospitals have bone banks. Are these sometimes used to provide bone for fusions?

Yes, occasionally they are, when too much bone is required to take it all from the patient himself. As long as enough can be obtained from a suitable donor site, however, the patient's own bone is preferred, since it is never rejected by the body and is thought to have the potential to stimulate new bone growth. Bone bank bone, on the other hand, has no such potential but merely serves as a scaffold that allows the body's own bone-forming cells to grow in and bridge adjacent vertebrae.

How long does it take to recover from a typical fusion?

Depending on the extent of the fusion I will recommend you stay in your hospital bed for a few days to a week or more, and to keep you immobile I will fit you with a corset or brace. For a day or two you may not be able to get up without help from the nurses and physical therapists. Once you get over your weakness and soreness and can walk comfortably, I will let you go home.

I won't pretend that you'll have an easy time of it for those first few days. Besides the pain and soreness from the fusion, you will have the added discomfort of the incision in the pelvis where the bone was taken out. In fact the donor site may go on being sore long after the fusion has healed.

Once you get home, you should spend at least three to four months avoiding movements that could endanger the fusion – no prolonged sitting, no heavy lifting, no vigorous bending, no violent twisting. You need that period of limited activity to give the graft a chance to become fully incorporated. It may take up to six months for you to feel the full benefit of the fusion – that is, to recover completely from your original symptoms and your post-operative discomfort.

Is there some certain way of knowing when a fusion has completely taken?

Not easily. Plain X-ray can give a very misleading impression, and even the CT may be difficult to interpret. X-rays taken with the spine bent forward and backward may be helpful, but usually the success or failure of the fusion is judged according to the patient's clinical response. However, some surgeons have gone as far as to suggest that if severe, disabling symptoms persist, the only way to tell whether a fusion is solid is to open up the back and look at it.

You may find yourself among the group who get almost immediate pain relief. This is a puzzling phenomenon, and no one understands fully how such a rapid response can take place. After all, the surgeon has not actually grafted one bone to another; he has merely created the conditions under which nature will gradually produce a fusion. Yet many patients will feel a change in their symptoms right after surgery. The old intolerable pain has been replaced by a new discomfort that seems certain to disappear.

How do you think those speedy recoveries can be explained?

I can only speculate, but I believe the most important factor is the temporary reduction in movement that comes from wedging bone between the vertebral bodies and into the facet joints, or from linking the bones together with metal plates. After all, reduced mobility of the affected segment is the ultimate goal of fusion. Another factor is how severely the patient's activities are restricted. If you just put on a brace and stay in bed, your back has a good chance of becoming pain free as long as you remain that way. I have noticed, too, that with some patients, extensive surgery destroys the nerve supply to the muscles of the back. For several months, those muscles are incapable of going into spasm. At least temporarily, the patient will have some relief from muscular pain. There's also an emotional factor: having been through a big operation, the patient probably tends, subconsciously or otherwise, to minimize any residual pain. Of course, that emotional factor can work in just the opposite way; a sudden back spasm or twinge of leg pain may produce acute anxiety.

But the short-term effects are different from the permanent pain relief you hope the fusion will achieve?

Yes. In a successful fusion, you'll get lasting pain relief because a solid bar of bone guarantees there is no movement.

Can spinal fusion lead to specific complications?

Yes, it can. Loss of movement at one level puts extra stress on the discs and joints above and below. With time, a few patients will develop new trouble at a different location and start the cycle all over again.

In rare instances, fusion outside the spinal canal will cause the bone inside to produce new growth that narrows the tunnel. This leads to spinal stenosis and nerve-root compression that may require further surgery.

More often, the complications are not so serious or long-lasting. For example, a fusion patient may become too dependent on his back brace, and the doctor will have difficulty weaning him away from it. To do so, the doctor will prescribe a rigid schedule: go without the brace for one hour a day for one week, then two hours a day the second week, and so on. The patient is instructed to put the brace back on after the prescribed time, whether or not he feels the need for it. Knowing he'll soon be wearing the brace again, he's unlikely to panic without it. Meanwhile, the act of wearing the brace becomes dissociated from the sense of need, and the patient begins to feel confident that his back is regaining its normal stability.

What about the recovery period at home? Do you have a standard list of do's and don'ts for patients recuperating from decompression or fusion surgery?

As you know by now, I am not generally inclined to write hard and fast rules for my patients, but there are some necessary cautions and a few complications I always mention, on the principle that forewarned is forearmed.

The most important points cover daily living habits. For the first few weeks, be conscious of your body movements and posture. Sit, lift, turn, and bend with moderation. After the fourth day, you can wash the area of the incision, as long as you pat the wound dry, but because tub bathing requires sitting in a poor position, you're better off under a shower.

I have found an early return to regular exercise remarkably helpful. With proper supervision some patients can begin to work out within two weeks of surgery. Everyone should be given an exercise routine before the end of the second month. Surgeons sometimes neglect this aspect of post-operative management because they expect the physical therapist to set it up. The physical therapist, on the other hand, is often reluctant to start such a program without the surgeon's approval. As the person with the most to gain, the patient mustn't be afraid to ask how soon exercise can be started.

Is convalescence likely to be a painful period?

Not as a rule, but a few unpleasant things can happen to make you fear the surgery has failed and your old trouble is still with you. The post-operative pain is more likely to arise from other causes, and you'll be better off knowing about them because unexpected pain produces fear, which greatly aggravates the problem. You may develop a cramp or troublesome tingling feelings in your leg where the pain used to be, because the involved nerve is still irritable and inclined to reproduce the old symptoms. The amount of discomfort will vary according to several factors, including the amount of pressure there was on the nerve before surgery, how long that pressure had existed, how much inflammation was present, and how much force the surgeon had to use to retract the nerve to get at the location of the trouble. Remember, your symptoms are only "leftovers," and now that the irritation has been removed the nerve will begin to recover.

Another possible complication, which is less likely and usually less serious than you may suppose, is a vascular condition called phlebitis. Lying on a special frame or in a "knee-chest" position during surgery may interfere with the flow of blood in the veins of the legs. The problem can be aggravated if you are required to remain in bed after surgery. Although the term phlebitis means inflammation of the veins, the real problem is the small blood clots that form at the sites of inflammation. These small clots may lead to the formation of larger clots that can break loose and travel up the vein. One of these mobile clots, now known as an embolus, may lodge in the lung, causing a condition called pulmonary embolism. This, in turn, can put the affected area of the lung out of commission, although even that is not a serious matter if the area is small.

If phlebitis does occur, what can you do about it?

The leg pain from the local inflammation can be treated with elastic support stockings, rest, and elevation of the affected leg. Some doctors use anti-inflammatory medication, and anti-coagulants which will stop the clots from forming. In fact, for certain types of back surgery, it has become routine to use anti-embolic elastic stockings during the operation and to administer an anti-coagulant, as preventive measures. The incidence of phlebitis, a rare complication to begin with, has been further reduced by these precautions.

Because they may have been told about phlebitis by their doctors, or heard about it from friends, many patients worry about this problem. Fortunately, most people who fear they have developed phlebitis after surgery are in fact suffering temporarily from conditions that need cause no concern. For instance, if you had surgery for disc pressure on the nerve that supplies your calf muscles, cramps may recur during the healing period, causing temporary soreness. Or if you lie in bed for several days – and this is true whether you've had surgery or not – you'll find your leg muscles will complain when you try to get up. Both these conditions can be mistaken for phlebitis. The correct diagnosis should be made after careful physical examination, and in some cases after specific blood flow and isotope studies.

Are there other problems likely to occur during convalescence?

You may have a difficult time getting back to normal living, both for physical and psychological reasons. It can take you a while before you feel like eating normally. Right after the operation you may have no appetite at all. Major spinal surgery often shuts down the gastro-intestinal tract for a few days. If you eat during that period the food doesn't go far; it just lies there and gives you stomach cramps. Even when you're home again you may take some time to get your old appetite back.

But while accepting the limitations mentioned so far, you should be trying to return to your customary living habits as soon as you can. Don't be shy, for instance, about asking your doctor when you can resume sexual intercourse. Your doctor has heard that question before and will be quite prepared to give you specific advice. As a general rule, the answer is: "The sooner the better."

Recovering from surgery is really quite an art – but an art most people can master with ease. Apart from a few basics, there are no techniques that suit everybody, and there's plenty of room for individual style and judgment. I well remember one patient of mine, the owner of a clothing store, who came out of hospital after disc surgery late in November. Two weeks later, I dropped by his store, and there he was, standing cheerfully behind the counter with one foot up on a block of wood. Perhaps he should have been resting at home, but he couldn't bear being away from the business during the Christmas rush.

I wish I could have pointed him out to another man I operated on for the same problem. This patient was obviously brought up in a family that doted on high drama. Two days after he came out of the operating room, I visited him at the hospital, and there he lay, hands folded over his chest in funereal repose, while a dozen ashen-faced relatives sat around the room, whispering solemnly to one another. If Central Casting had been looking for a convincing corpse, I could have steered them to a prime candidate. Of course, he didn't die but went home instead, with the entourage of mourners in tow, and spent at least three months playing out his role as the family's critically disabled convalescent.

If you want to get off to a good start at home, resolve not to play invalid or load your spouse and family with guilt if they decline to cater to your every whim. Certainly you want them to be aware of what you're going through and what you are up against, but it won't help anyone, least of all yourself, to overstate your difficulties or limitations.

It would be a mistake to underestimate the influence that interpersonal relations can have on your physical well-being. I had one woman patient whose symptoms during her time in hospital were clearly aggravated by her husband. Whenever he was around, she lost her ability to walk and suffered excruciating pain. The moment he went away, she returned to normal.

By all means, follow the basic rules of good physical care throughout the early weeks of convalescence. But never ignore the psychological side. Nothing can help you recover more swiftly or more completely than a positive attitude on your part and a readiness on the part of those around you to help you return to your normal style of living.

What about the long-term results of neck and back surgery?

Once you get a good result it tends to stay good. There is some natural wear and tear, of course, and both the site of the surgery and the adjacent levels remain slightly more vulnerable. But in a recent study of the long-term results of spine surgery, over 95 percent of the patients felt satisfied with the outcome, and only 15 to 20 percent showed signs of new trouble that might require further treatment.

What do you see in the future for patients needing a back operation?

There are some amazing possibilities, and the technology for most of them already exists. Outpatients might be sent through a CT scan and a magnetic resonance imaging (MRI) machine that could locate, analyze, and diagnose the surgical problem. Under local anesthesia the patient could undergo an automated discotomy with

X-ray control using a power cutting tool introduced through a large needle in the back. Somatosensory evoked potentials (SEP) would tell the operator when enough nucleus had been removed to relieve the nerve pressure. Through the same needle the hollow disc center could then be filled with a mixture of bone and biological glue to create an immediate solid fusion. The whole experience might eventually become as routine and brief as a visit to the dentist.

I'm sure doctors of the future will marvel at how we ever managed to produce *any* satisfactory results with our primitive twentieth-century equipment.

13. If You're Thinking of Going to Court...

Like many other specialists, I devote a certain amount of my professional time to legal cases, examining accident victims whose injuries fall within the range of my work as an orthopedic surgeon.

Most of these patients come to me on referral from lawyers, either their own or those on the opposing side. A few come from insurance companies who also want to determine the effects of the accident and the extent of disability.

While such evaluations are necessary, I am disturbed by the way they and the other steps in litigation often hamper accident victims in their recovery. Unavoidably, the extensive legal preparation and the trial itself force patients to relive a bad experience, perhaps reviving dormant pain and prolonging the present condition. Even worse, the situation compels them to focus constantly on remaining symptoms and other negative aspects of their condition.

That increased awareness of pain and disability is, of course, exactly opposite to the attitude a person should adopt if he wants to recover swiftly from injury and return to normal living. Clearly, a preoccupation with the problem is one important step in the development of the chronic pain syndrome which, as we have seen, is a behavioral disease from which some people never recover.

The motives for going to court are understandable. We all like to see justice done – to see the guilty called to account and their victims compensated for all losses and suffering. And, of course, with the increasing size of awards handed down by our courts these days, the prospects of a successful lawsuit are becoming more and more attractive.

After years of direct experience with thousands of accident victims, however, I have concluded that the financial rewards of personal injury litigation are seldom worth the price. This is a message many patients would rather not hear – especially those who are already committed to legal action – but I believe it needs to be said.

I have included in this chapter not only some practical tips for accident victims who decide to sue, but also – and more important, I think – some observations on the destructive side effects of litigation. I hope readers will consider my arguments and form realistic opinions before they have reason to become embroiled in a personal injury lawsuit, exposing themselves to the emotional stress and family pressure that so often propel an accident victim into court.

Suppose I'm to have a medical examination for a lawsuit. Do you have any advice?

There are two basic points. First, try to answer the doctor's questions as factually and concisely as you can. Since the information you provide will go into a report to be read by many other people, and may also be presented in court as verbal evidence that is subject to cross-examination, you should take special care to make yourself clearly understood. Keep in mind that the doctor is interested primarily in your mental and physical condition. This will include the mechanism of your injury but it has nothing to do with the potential liability. For example, it's important for you to describe the direction of impact in a motor vehicle collision, but it doesn't matter to the doctor who had the right of way or whether the other driver had been drinking.

Second, try to describe your condition accurately in words that are not overly dramatic or emotionally charged. For example, it's not helpful to say, "Whenever I try to move, an excruciating pain shoots all over my body." Instead, be as specific as you can: "Usually, the pain is worse when I try to walk, and it seems to be mostly down my right leg."

It might be useful to make some notes about your symptoms and how they have changed since the accident. But keep the descriptions brief; jot things down in point form.

It's not always that easy to describe your own back pain, especially in a few words.

You're right – it isn't. But the doctor is trained to help you by asking specific questions that are easy to answer. Is the pain steady or throbbing? Does it feel sharp or dull? Is the pain associated with burning or tingling sensations? These are the types of standard questions doctors use in helping patients describe their symptoms. Which reminds me of a conversation I overhead when I was a medical student. One of my teachers had just come back from a vacation abroad, and another doctor wanted to hear about it. But he didn't just ask, "How was your trip?" He asked, "Was the weather hot or cold? Was it wet or dry? Was the tour interesting or disappointing?" And so on. And in response to each question, my clinician was solemnly choosing the appropriate answer. I'm sure they never realized that, out of force of habit, one doctor was conducting a professional inquiry into the other doctor's vacation.

In a medical examination, this style of questioning helps you avoid offering descriptions that are unrealistic and therefore unhelpful. In their sincere attempt to convey the full magnitude and intensity of the problem, some patients will tell me, "It feels exactly like I've been stabbed with a red-hot spear" or "It feels just like I've been kicked by an elephant." I sympathize with anyone suffering that amount of pain, but those sorts of descriptions don't help me define the problem, since I've never been stabbed with a red-hot spear or kicked by an elephant. It isn't that I don't understand the meaning of the comparisons but they give me nothing I can write down and use in my report.

It must be difficult to prepare a report when you believe the patient is deliberately exaggerating for effect.

It is. And it's even worse when the patient, consciously or otherwise, seems to be hiding the truth. For instance, I remember one case where four people, injured while riding in the back seat of a car, insisted they had all been wearing seat belts, which are compulsory in Ontario. Their story was difficult to believe, since the back seat of the car was equipped with only three belts. Someone had to be wrong.

In reporting a case like that, I would write, "The patient says he was wearing a seat belt," not just "the patient was wearing a seat belt." In other words, I would record the patient's claim in a non-judgmental phrase, without accepting his statement as fact.

I can understand why the victim's own lawyer wants your report. Are you ever asked to examine a patient sent by a lawyer representing the opposing side?

Yes, it happens frequently. A personal injury victim involved in litigation is legally obliged to submit to an examination by a doctor selected by the other side. This is generally referred to as an IME, "independent medical examination." Obviously the patient can feel threatened by this situation and in rare instances may even refuse to answer the doctor's questions during the assessment.

What do you do if someone refuses to tell you anything?

First I try to explain that my role is not to judge the case but only to determine the patient's medical condition. In most instances my report should be virtually the same as the one prepared by the patient's own doctor. If you asked me whether you should co-operate in that situation, I'd say yes, definitely. I think you'd be foolish to do otherwise, because your refusal could suggest you have something to hide. Besides, the IME is really just a second opinion on your problem from a designated expert in the field. That specialist might even find something significant that your own doctor missed. You will get a useful opinion only if you participate willingly in the examination.

When a patient absolutely refuses, I simply report that I conducted the examination but could not elicit all the information I wanted because the person declined to co-operate. I don't imagine it helps their case if this fact is brought out in court, but that's not my concern.

If you had examined me for litigation, would you be willing to tell me what you intend to say in your report?

As a rule, I'm very open about my opinion. I believe you should know as much about your problem as you can. And I don't think it matters whether you hear it from your own doctor or the one who examines you for the other side. Besides, once the reports are prepared and filed with the court, they become public record and anyone can read them.

Do you have any special advice about the way I should handle myself in court?

Your lawyer will give you a more thorough briefing, but I can tell you a few things I've learned from my experience as an expert witness. The most important thing is also the simplest: tell the truth. Don't try to improve your case by coloring your answers or holding back relevant facts. If you are trying to establish that you have a serious injury, nobody will expect you to minimize your suffering; but if you present the facts in a balanced way, the court is more likely to believe you. For instance, if you have been able to do certain physical things in spite of your pain, I suggest you say so right from the start. Don't leave it for the other side to introduce the evidence in a way that will cause embarrassment for you or your doctor.

I was once embarrassed in the witness box when I learned for the first time that my patient, whose disability I had just described in considerable detail, was in fact well enough to be working seven days a week. He was putting in five days a week as a taxi driver and making a long trip out of town every weekend to work as a ski instructor. The man had carefully avoided telling me this, and so had his lawyer. Of course when the defendant's lawyer presented these facts and asked me whether they would alter my assessment of the man's disability, I naturally admitted they would. I wasn't surprised or, I admit, disappointed when the plaintiff lost his case.

I have also learned that if you are asked a question you don't fully understand, you shouldn't be afraid to get clarification before answering. No one should object if you ask the lawyer to repeat the question. To avoid confusion you might rephrase it in your own words before you respond.

Don't pretend to know things that are outside your knowledge or experience, such as the speed of the approaching car you glimpsed for only a second. That last bit of advice is something I heed myself, as an expert witness. Sometimes on the stand I am asked to give an opinion about something I just don't know. For example, I might be asked to compare the victim's pain before and after a second accident that aggravated his original injuries. Since pain is a totally subjective experience that defies direct measurement, there is no way to answer that question with any degree of accuracy. In such a situation I would explain my reasons and decline to speculate.

Do you think many patients deliberately lie about their disability for personal gain?

True malingering is rare. Very few people invent all their symptoms just to collect money in court. Most patients accused of malingering are probably not lying as much as exaggerating. They're afraid that if they aren't blatant enough about their pain the examiner won't fully appreciate that there is something wrong. I think we're all inclined to cope with the same injury in different ways, depending on the situation. Suppose you were a member of a wedding party and you twisted your ankle on the way into the church. Wouldn't you do your best to disguise your pain and injury throughout the ceremony? But if that same twisted ankle needed examining in the course of a lawsuit, surely you would limp into the doctor's office. Yet it would hardly be fair to say you were faking your injury to increase your chances in court.

Of course, there are exceptions. As a surgical resident I examined a man with back pain who I was sure had no real problem and was trying to fool me. But after I discharged him from the emergency room I had second thoughts, and so I slipped out a side entrance to follow him up the street. I must have been quite a sight in my white suit hiding behind parked cars and peering around the corners of buildings. However, he never saw me, and after two or three blocks, sure enough, his limp disappeared and he began to walk normally.

Besides following someone out of your office, how can you tell if a patient isn't being honest with you about his condition?

Like all experienced back examiners, I have developed physical tests that are designed to weed out people who are consciously exaggerating their symptoms. The results tell me whether the person is reporting honestly.

Even if someone takes the trouble to discover these techniques, many of my tests require movements that simply can't be faked. Here's one example. Suppose you describe weakness of your ankle that causes you to walk with a limp. I will ask you to sit in a chair with both feet flat on the floor. Next I will have you raise your forefoot on the affected side while keeping the heel of that foot on the floor. Now I squat in front of you, place one hand over the instep of your foot, and ask you to maintain your position against the downward pressure of my hand. If you have a true muscular weakness, your foot will yield smoothly until it's flat on the floor. But if your power is normal and you are trying to fool me, the forefoot won't sink smoothly; instead, it will descend unevenly in little "cogwheel" steps that tell me you're faking. The interesting thing is that even with practice, you can never develop the smooth muscular release that denotes true weakness, and so the test works even if you know all about it.

I'm careful not to rely on just one or two such examinations. I use several, and they all have to produce consistent results. Also, I often test the same condition in three or four different ways, without the patient's realizing it. For instance, if a patient complains of neck pain and exhibits a greatly reduced range of movement, I sometimes stand behind him and start talking. It's remarkable to watch someone who can't move his neck at all during the examination turn his head around quite comfortably to look at me when I speak. People whose complaints are genuine won't react that way.

Have you found that accident victims involved in litigation exaggerate their pain more than other patients?

In many cases they do. And that exaggeration can become a problem in itself. I think the extent of the behavior depends on what patients expect from the doctor and what they believe they have to do to get him to meet those expectations.

Most of us are skeptical about those who go to court seeking large awards for their pain and suffering. It's easy to assume that accident victims merely suffer until their cases are settled satisfactorily, and that once they collect a big award, their health suddenly improves.

Certainly most lawyers and doctors can recall one or two victims who had a "miraculous" improvement once they received a large financial settlement. But if you consider the thousands of personal injury actions initiated each year, you will find that such "miracles" are exceptions rather than the rule.

When a person decides whether or not to enter into a lawsuit over his injuries, he may well be deciding, without realizing it, whether to set out on the road to recovery or to assume the role of a suffering litigant for years to come.

Are you saying that all accident victims who take legal action will be trapped in the role of an injured person?

No, not always, but it does happen far too often. To achieve what he sees as a just settlement, the accident victim may concentrate on his disability until it becomes an obsession. He will tend to focus on his symptoms and magnify or at least sustain the pain in order to further his case. Soon, he is thinking and talking about little else. He becomes a "professional victim" whose disability affects every aspect of his life, destroying his ability to work and straining his relationships with family and friends.

Often a marriage suffers badly. Like patients with the chronic pain syndrome, people emotionally involved in injury litigation can experience sexual problems brought on by the psychological strain and the preoccupation with their health. It's difficult for a worried mind to become sexually aroused. As a "professional victim," a man may be impotent or a woman unresponsive for reasons that do not stem directly from the disability or any physical impairment of sexual function.

When you consider what these changes in personality can mean to the way the person will live, you have to ask whether any amount of money awarded in court can be worth the price. Those problems will not happen to everyone, but you should be aware of the possibility when you choose to sue over a personal injury.

As you realize by now, the psychology of prolonged litigation disability is much the same as that of the chronic pain syndrome, and in fact some accident victims make the unfortunate transition into CPS. Partly because of the way the legal process holds their recovery in abeyance during the usually lengthy process, these people maintain the expected pattern of behavior to the point where it becomes permanent.

It strikes me there is something wrong with a system that allows such a thing to happen.

It's easy for some professionals to criticize "the system." But we are very much part of that system and have to take responsibility for the way it works. There are many advantages to the adversarial approach in law, and I am not suggesting we change the method. But every lawyer and doctor involved on either side of a personal injury action has an ethical obligation to settle the matter as fairly and as rapidly as possible to help the patient get on with his or her life. Yet it would be naive to suggest that there are no incentives for us to prolong an accident victim's recovery. If a case is settled quickly and inexpensively, there are no substantial legal fees. And there are fewer charges for conducting medical examinations and writing depositions. Many delays are unavoidable; the courts are overburdened. But prolonging the litigation also has significant financial benefits for the law firm or medical practice.

In some instances a doctor may unwittingly retard the process for fear of being wrong and jeopardizing the case. He may say, "I can't be sure yet – let me see the patient again in a year's time." A request like that means nobody is going to settle for at least a year, and meanwhile the patient must keep on feeling pain. Yet, medically, there's no basis for it. Without the pressure of providing a medical-legal opinion, no competent doctor would wait twelve months before deciding on a course of treatment or giving the patient some idea of what to expect.

And I suppose that if the patient has already decided to stay home from work to avoid jeopardizing his case, that postponement will reinforce his decision.

That's right – and it's an extremely important point. Usually, the best way to recover swiftly from an accident is to return to work and resume all other normal activities as soon as possible.

But suppose, as the accident victim, I'm still in pain?

My advice may, at first, sound cold and uncaring, but I would still say: get back on the job, pain and all, and do your best to stop behaving like a disabled person. How you see yourself, or more precisely how the legal action *forces* you to see yourself, is critical. The more you think you can achieve the more you will be able to do. Of course, the speed of your return to work will depend in part on the nature of your job. You may have to wait longer before getting back to heavy construction work than to an office job. But resuming your regular employment is great for your self-image, and there is no medical basis for arguing that an early return to work will harm you. It may increase your pain temporarily, but it will not physically damage you or prevent your ultimate recovery.

Consider whether you'd rather put up with a little extra backache on the job while you get better or face the prospect of months or even years of suffering and disability that must be endured before the litigation is settled. Until recently the seriousness of that enforced delay in recovery wasn't fully appreciated. But new studies are changing our understanding. In one study of ninety-nine people who filed suits over injuries they suffered in industrial or car accidents, thirty-three were found to have returned to work before their cases were settled. Of the other sixty-six, only nine were found to have returned to work within sixteen months after settlement.

Isn't it likely that many of the remaining fifty-seven patients just needed more time to recover and would return to work later?

No, I'm afraid that's not likely. As we have found from other studies and experience, if you don't return to your job within two years after your back injury, chances are you never will. You may work at something light and inconsequential, perhaps part time, but you are most unlikely to return permanently to your regular employment. On the other hand, it was found that when a group of accident victims got the help they needed to physically overcome their injuries and develop a healthy pattern of behavior, 70 percent of them returned to work before their litigation was settled. In other words, litigation doesn't necessarily deter most people from going back to work if they are properly treated, if they want to go back, and if there is a job waiting for them.

Does the prospect of a large settlement have any influence on the person's inclination to sue or file a claim for disability?

Yes, it appears to. One study has shown that in jurisdictions where the average compensation award amounts to more than 55 percent of the pre-injury net income, the number of claims increases drastically. Some people even take this opportunity to leave the work force permanently. It's bad enough to be a disabled person, without becoming a prematurely retired disabled person. Retirement can be a happy state if it is planned and carried out willingly, with a sense of purpose. But under these circumstances, it's a dismal and wasteful way to spend the rest of your life.

What about the accident victim who says, "Sure, I'll go back to work later, but I'd be a sucker to make any move until I get the big settlement I deserve"?

Unfortunately, a few people do concentrate on the money. I had one patient who had been injured in two accidents. Right after the second one, she declared she had made a serious mistake settling her first claim too soon – and by that she meant too cheaply. Now she was determined to collect enough from the second injury to make up for that earlier deficiency. There was very little logic in her approach, and I knew with that attitude she had no chance of making another rapid recovery. But the amount of her previous award would have no bearing on the size of her second settlement (if she won her case). The new award, if any, would be based entirely on the minor injuries caused by the more recent accident. After the legal fees and disbursements were deducted, her potential financial gain would be modest. More important, no financial award of any size would compensate for the way her spiteful approach was distorting her personality and lifestyle.

Fortunately, that woman was not typical of the injured people I normally see. In my experience, few are that calculating. Initially, at least, most accident victims just want to return to work and get on with their lives. But if they embark on litigation, they take on a commitment they feel they must keep. Later, as the action drags on and on, their physical condition deteriorates and they lose their job skills, their self-discipline, their work habits, and their motivation. They feel like strangers to their old colleagues or workmates. By then it's too late to get back on the job.

A friend of mine who went to court over an injury in a car accident was encouraged to keep a daily record of how she felt. Is that helpful to the doctor or lawyer?

I would rather you asked whether it's helpful to the patient. Then my answer would be: that depends on why the person is keeping the "pain journal," as it's commonly called. That daily log is useful if it is kept as part of a treatment program designed to help the patient recover from the injury and conquer the disability. The person will find it encouraging to look back and see how function is being restored while the discomfort and pain are receding.

It's quite a different thing, however, to keep a pain journal for legal purposes. Some lawyers recommend it to their clients, but medically I consider it a harmful practice when there is no accompanying therapy. The diary becomes nothing more than a daily record of misery that encourages the victim to focus his attention on his pain. That approach may help win court cases but it certainly doesn't help people get well.

It can be difficult to write a journal that satisfies both your doctor and your lawyer. While your doctor will be hoping to see a record of steady recovery, for the sake of the litigation your lawyer will want it to show a pattern of continuing disability. I recommend you use the pain journal as an aid to getting well, not to staying sick. Keep the litigation secondary in your mind and concentrate on recovering. Everyone's goal should be a rapid and complete return to a normal lifestyle and the prompt settlement of the lawsuit.

Have you found that a family's support can help the patient keep those priorities straight?

Some families provide positive encouragement that helps hasten the patient's return to normal life. But others unconsciously reinforce the harmful reactions that delay recovery.

If there are grounds for a lawsuit, a family may rally around the victim – "Mother's been hurt, and we will see to it that the person responsible pays for her injury." Although everyone's intentions are the best, the last thing Mother may need, for her own good, is the added stress of becoming a litigant. But there are no pressures stronger than those imposed by a person's own family. After all, the family has already done so much. They have arranged the medical care, visited Mother in the hospital, and begun tending her at home. In a situation like this, the family members have developed their own expectations, and everyone – Mother included – tends to react accordingly. Now they've hired a lawyer to see that justice is done. Mother can hardly turn around at this point and say, "Never mind, I don't want to sue anyone. I'm going to be fine."

Declining to go along with the family could be the smartest thing Mother ever did – but how many of us could do it?

And so, unwittingly, the family creates and reinforces the patient's new self-image as a disabled person, smothering the victim with over-protection and receiving, in response, the sad compliment of child-like dependence.

To cope with the new stress of a protracted legal action and the accompanying lengthy period of disability, the family not only provides increased support but also restructures itself, forming new relationships that are ostensibly benign, temporary, and helpful. In truth, they will change the lives of all those involved. The formerly passive spouse suddenly takes charge, and the once-dominant mate, as victim, meekly complies. Or Big Sister, once eager to further her career by handling a full-time job and a heavy course at night school, abruptly quits both to stay home and look after Poor Mother. What loving family could do less, especially now that the Disabled One is facing the strange and frightening obstacles of litigation?

The problem becomes even more complex when two or more family members are injured in the same accident. I once examined a mother, father, and three children, all involved in a lawsuit over a rear-end collision. No one had been seriously hurt, physically, but the ensuing legal battle had a devastating effect on the structure of the family. The suit became their principal family business. Unconsciously, everyone was reluctant to let the team down by getting better. And no one did.

With the inception of personal injury litigation we may begin a self-perpetuating situation that can alter the lives of all who buy into it. As one litigant's spouse said with rare insight, "It would take a miracle for us to be like we used to be."

Is there something the injured person, or the family, can do from the outset to avoid that trap?

Yes. With sound legal advice and medical support, the accident victim and the family should agree from the start to share just one objective: getting everyone back to normal living as soon as possible. And if that means putting up with some temporary pain, or passing up the "opportunity" to pursue a supposedly rewarding lawsuit, so be it.

14. A NEW APPROACH TO HELPFUL EXERCISE

People often ask me, "What's new in back care?" And, just as often, I surprise them by answering, "Exercise!"

Of course, I don't mean I have just discovered that proper exercise is useful in preventing back pain. I've been spreading that message for years. But we are now beginning to understand that exercise can also help to relieve the pain of a subsiding attack and so can assist in short-term recovery. Meanwhile, doctors and physical therapists who specialize in back care are achieving significant discoveries and developments to make back exercises more effective than ever.

For my part, in the seven years since I wrote *The Back Doctor*, I have been continually reassessing and refining the exercise routines I recommend to my patients and to classes at the Canadian Back Institute (formerly the Canadian Back Education Units). While I have found nothing to suggest that those earlier workouts were anything but helpful, I have devised ways of improving the program by modifying some exercises and emphasizing the importance of others.

I have come to appreciate more fully the value of combining two complementary types of exercise – flexion (forward bending) and extension (backward bending) – and I have learned from clinical experience that for most patients the best program consists of a comfortable balance between the two. This evolution in my thinking means, among other things, that although I included extension exercises in *The Back Doctor*, I now place greater emphasis on them. I also focus more attention on exercises that stretch the back muscles and put the small joints through a range of movement.

Readers familiar with the exercises contained in *The Back Doctor* will see both similarities and differences in the routines presented here. Perhaps the first new thing they will notice is the way the presentation makes clear distinctions between flexion and extension and between stretching and strengthening. While such valuable old standbys as the sit-up are inevitably included, they are presented in a fresh context that reflects my new approach.

Since my philosophy of back care remains unchanged, people who are comfortable with the exercises I favored in my earlier book should feel equally at ease with those they find here. My view that each person must bear the ultimate responsibility for the care of his or her own back applies especially to exercise. It's up to each of us to find, and practice, the routines that suit our individual situations. After all, we come in various shapes and sizes, with individual muscular strengths and weaknesses, differing attitudes towards exercise, and unique personal habits and lifestyles.

No arbitrary set of exercises could possibly fill the bill for everyone who reads this book. What I offer here, then, is not a prescription but a list of recommendations, an assortment of routines from which you, as a backache sufferer, can choose in creating your own custom-made exercise program, subject only to certain limitations I mention along the way. If you are using exercises from *The Back Doctor* and they're working, I suggest you continue them and perhaps try a few I've presented here.

On the other hand, if the idea of back exercise is new to you, you will want to look over the possibilities and experiment with several routines that apply to your situation before you create your permanent repertoire. You can make a more intelligent choice if you understand which form of back pain you have – Type One, Two, Three, or Four – but, even then, you may have to continue your search for exercises to accommodate the special needs of your situation. Think of yourself as a watchman, new on the job, equipped with a huge ring of keys. Several are necessary to unlock the doors along the passages where you want to go; but only by trial and error will you find the right assortment.

The choices shouldn't be hard to make on your own, but if you are already seeing a doctor or physical therapist, you might like to take this book along and ask for comments and suggestions about the program that would suit you best.

While the exercises you find here bear my stamp of approval and that of the Canadian Back Institute, they are not my inventions, and I make no claim about their being original, much less uniquely mine. But whether you think of them as Dr. Hamilton Hall's exercises or not, I suggest you make some of them your own. I think you will find them helpful, and you can be sure that if you do them as directed, they won't harm your back or any other part of your body.

My advice, then, is to move carefully but confidently. It's quite likely that within these next pages you can find a lasting solution to your back problem.

I'm anxious to get started on an exercise program to get rid of my back pain, but I'd like to know how long I'll have to keep at it.

There's no time limit. As long as you want the benefit to continue, you'll have to keep on with your exercises. Otherwise, you'll be making the mistake often made by people who want to lose weight. They attend special classes and go on special diets until they've shed the pounds they want to get rid of. Then they go right back to their old eating habits. And we all know what happens to their waistlines after that.

But you're suggesting a lifelong commitment! Do you really mean I have to do my exercises every day for the rest of my life?

Why not? You put your clothes on every day, don't you? And brush your teeth and comb your hair? What's the difference? We're talking about an additional allotment of ten or twelve minutes a day – probably less time than you spend showering and toweling yourself dry. You're quite accustomed to performing those other simple tasks of personal care, and if you think of your exercises as just one extra item, no more difficult or complicated than the rest, you won't find it hard to fit them into your life. It is the main reason I keep the exercise program short and simple. The truth is, that if people find their daily exercises don't take long, they are more likely to continue with them. On the other hand, if you look upon your exercises as something to be dreaded, you'll eventually give up on them and lose a lot of the gains you've made.

Are you saying that once I get started, I'll be in trouble if I quit?

You won't be worse off than you were before you started exercising, but many people who have begun a back exercise program and then neglected it have told me their pain returned when they stopped. And the cause-and-effect relationship seems evident, since they also say that once they started their exercises again, the pain subsided. Part of the problem in recognizing the value of exercises is the length of time they require to produce results and the gradual way in which they improve the situation in terms of reduced severity of pain and accelerated rate of recovery. You won't feel any change immediately, and no patient ever says, "I remember that after I had been exercising for exactly six months, I got up one wonderful Thursday morning and my back pain had disappeared." If you're tempted to quit, you might remind yourself of how much more fun you have when your back is in good shape and you can enjoy your favorite activities.

I'm interested in getting into an exercise class for general fitness. Should I do that if my doctor has told me to take care of my back?

Yes, you can safely take part in almost any general exercise program if you carefully pick and choose the exercises you do. Talk it over with the instructor beforehand and discuss any exercises you might want to avoid. Your decision of course depends mainly on the type of back or neck pain you have. For example, if you have discogenic pain, which I call Type Two, you may find that sit-ups are painful, and you will want to avoid them and work out some substitutes.

If you have neck pain referred between your shoulder blades, a program specifically designed to strengthen the shoulder muscles, using free weights or an exercise machine, may provide you with the only source of lasting relief.

You may want to postpone your enrollment in a class until you have developed your own back or neck exercise routine. By then you'll have a better understanding of which exercises are painful for you and which are all right.

You said earlier there are certain aerobic routines that aren't good for your back. What substitutes do you suggest?

Among the exercises that have caused the most trouble for back patients are the "high-bounce" aerobics – that is, those where you jump up and down violently. It's possible to give your heart and lungs the equivalent workout by performing a shuffling movement that is rapid but not as violent. Standing in one spot, quickly slide your feet forward and backward alternately, letting the soles of your feet graze the floor with each stride.

Or, to use another example, you can stimulate your heart and lungs with the familiar arm-raising exercise – standing with your arms at your sides and rapidly raising them to shoulder height, then dropping them back again – without the stride-jumping that is usually part of that routine.

Are there any exercises you never recommend because they irritate muscles or joints without providing much benefit?

Yes, I can think of two or three that everybody ought to avoid. One consists of rolling your head around and around in a circle from shoulder to shoulder. People do this imagining they are relaxing their neck muscles, but all they are doing in reality is making themselves feel dizzy, while the backward part of the roll compresses their neck joints. If you want to exercise your neck properly, I suggest you try the routines I will describe later.

Deep knee bends are another item on my forbidden list. They don't stretch or strengthen your leg or back muscles any better than half knee bends do, and they are far too hard on your knee joints. In the half knee bend, you should lower your body to the point where your thighs are parallel to the floor, as if you were seated in a chair. The half knee bend and its variation, an exercise called The Imaginary Chair, both appear on my list.

A third exercise to avoid – and the silliest one I can think of offhand – consists of lying on your back and forcefully flexing your spine so that your pelvis is above your head and your feet are kicking the ground over your shoulders. It was part of those old macho athletic training routines abandoned years ago by more enlightened instructors. The action offers no useful benefits and creates needless strain on the neck, back, and thighs. There was a time when training exercises in sports were based mostly on tradition. Coaches simply perpetuated the routines they had learned as players, many of them based on the premise that "if it hurts it's good for you." Today, trainers and coaches know otherwise. They have access to a large body of research in ergonomics – the study of human movement – and to various computerized and photographic devices that enable them to measure the benefits and effects of each specific exercise.

At the CBI we have rejected several traditional exercises, and reached new conclusions about several others. We have found, for instance, that one familiar routine, toe touching, has notable limitations. Traditionally, it was done with the legs straight and the feet together – a position that imposes considerable strain on your back but does nothing to strengthen your paraspinal muscles. Toe touching can be useful as a stretching exercise, but it should be done with care. Start with your feet comfortably apart and your arms at your sides. As you bend your trunk, let your arms swing loose. As long as your upper body drops down enough to stretch the muscles of your legs and hips, it doesn't really matter whether your hands actually reach far enough to touch your toes. Remember, you're supposed to be *exercising* your body, not torturing it.

Never begin this exercise by stretching your arms over your head and swinging them down to your feet in a giant arc. That's known as a "ballistic" movement – one that's sudden and violent and uses gravity and momentum rather than muscle activity to produce the result. It's far too vigorous for most people, especially those with low-back pain, and it adds nothing extra to stretch or strengthen the muscles.

Before I try to make my personal choices from your list of recommended exercises, can you give me some basic advice as to what I should be looking for?

In order to pick the back exercises that will be the most helpful for you, make sure you know what type of back trouble you have, what the exercises are supposed to do, and then make sure you are performing them properly. I'll be including that basic information along with my descriptions of the exercises themselves.

It's unfortunate how some fitness buffs waste their energy on misguided exercise. I talked to one patient who told me he was doing forty sit-ups a day to develop his belly muscles. I decided to test him. When I had him lie on his back with his knees bent and his feet unsupported, he was amazed that he could do only three sit-ups. Normally he hooked his feet under a couch, never realizing that the exercise, as he was doing it, was strengthening his thighs but doing virtually nothing for his stomach muscles. Experiences like that have taught me to be a little skeptical whenever a patient assures me that he or she is doing back exercises regularly. Usually I check with the supervising physical therapist or, as I did in this case, ask for a little demonstration. "Regularly" and "correctly" are not the same thing.

How do you decide which exercises to recommend for a particular patient?

The easiest way to understand the principles I apply is to think of your spine as not just one column but three: a front column consisting of discs alternating with the bone of the vertebral bodies; a back column consisting of a series of interlocking facet joints; and a middle column that is the canal containing the spinal cord and nerves. This is a handy concept because it enables us to identify the source of pain – that is, whether the symptoms originate mainly in the front column, the back column, or the middle column. Although the underlying cause (usually the ordinary wear and tear of normal aging) routinely involves more than one column, you will probably be feeling most of your pain in only one location. You should begin with the exercises designed to cope with the pain you feel.

Can you be more specific about the relationship between types of pain and the exercises that help control them?

Type One pain originates in the back or posterior column. Therefore, exercises are designed to open up that column and reduce the load on the small joints. For that reason, this condition calls primarily for flexion (forward bending) exercises.

Type Two pain is found in the anterior or forward column. And so the remedy calls for extension (backward bending) exercises that reduce pressure at the front.

However, since both Type One and Type Two problems can lead to a general stiffness, once the severe pain has subsided, everyone should do both flexion and extension exercises to limber up. Before choosing your routine, you should pay as much attention to the stage of your recovery as you do to the source of your pain.

Type Three pain originates in the middle column. In this case the problem is nerve pressure, which is not so readily relieved by exercise. Although Type Three pain comes from the nerve that is being pinched in the middle column, the culprit is usually a disc bulging backward from the front column. Flexion, which increases pressure within the disc, is not likely to be of any help at all, but often you can relieve the pain somewhat by extension (arching backward). According to physical therapist Robin McKenzie's theory, extension exercises shift the water content of the disc's nucleus forward to take pressure away from the nerve.

Type Four, spinal stenosis, is a narrowing of that middle column. Its pain can sometimes be relieved by altering the position of your back to increase the space available to the compressed nerves. This effect may be achieved through a series of flexion-stretching exercises. (Strengthening exercises are not particularly useful because the area is already rigid, so the increased stability produced by stronger muscles has no effect.) Bending forward tends to open up the posterior column where the exits for the nerves are located. If you manage to enlarge these exit holes, you may reduce the squeezing. Not all Type Four cases respond to exercise, however, especially if the affected passages are extremely narrow. And for reasons no one understands, the occasional Type Four pain will respond to extension-stretching exercises.

You keep distinguishing between stretching and strengthening exercises. How important is that difference?

Very important. Stretching exercises are designed to loosen tight joints or ligaments and allow a free range of movement. Without that normal range, back pain will persist just as pain may persist in any joint that has not been allowed to move for some time.

Strengthening provides muscle support for that increased movement which the joint might otherwise be unable to tolerate. Without this stability, the newly acquired mobility could cause pain by over-stretching the adjacent soft tissues.

It becomes obvious that both stretching and strengthening are necessary. In a proper exercise routine, the joints are stretched so that the range of movement can develop and then the muscles are strengthened to protect that range. Stretching without strengthening can lead to unnecessary pain as a result of poor support, whereas strengthening exercises alone seldom produce pain relief in stiff joints.

What exercises do you recommend for people with osteoporosis?

Exercise in general helps maintain bone calcium levels. Bone grows stronger in response to the load applied to it, and therefore exercise is an excellent way of stimulating your bones and maintaining their bulk. However, if you have, or suspect you have, bone that is already thin, you should be careful not to engage in too-vigorous exercise, particularly when it involves extreme flexion or extension that could cause fractures. If you are in your late middle age and you are embarking on a strenuous exercise program for the first time, you'd be wise to check with your doctor first.

The choice between flexion and extension exercises should still depend on the origin of your back pain. If you have no pain, a combination of both seems reasonable. Where osteoporosis is present, strengthening is more important than stretching.

I'd like to know more about the pelvic tilt. Is it still among the exercises you recommend?

I never considered the pelvic tilt an exercise, even though, for convenient reference, I listed it as such in *The Back Doctor*. The pelvic tilt is really a starting position for many of the flexion exercises and should be maintained during some of them to protect the discs from excessive load. It's possible, of course, to tilt the lower part of your pelvis forward while standing (ask any belly dancer), but for our exercises, the pelvic tilt is performed as you lie on your back with your knees bent and your feet flat on the floor. Without holding your breath, you tighten your abdominal muscles and flatten the small of your back against the floor by rolling your hips forward and contracting the muscles in your buttocks. You can raise your buttocks slightly but do not push with your feet. This may sound complicated, but it's really a very simple and gentle movement – one of those maneuvers that is (if I may twist a phrase) easier done than said.

Before the roles of stretching and extension exercises were emphasized, the pelvic tilt was considered the basic element in maintaining proper low-back posture. Although its role is now more specifically defined in relation to flexion-strengthening exercises, its general value has not been diminished.

*   *   *

So we come to my list of recommended exercises. Before we get into them, I have a few comments. The routine that will be right for you can come only from experimentation; there is no single pattern that will work for everyone or even for the same individual at all times. Consider both the source of your pain and the state of your recovery.

Keep your exercise period short (ten to fifteen minutes) so that it fits your day. Some people find that two daily sessions are helpful. The number of different exercises you do doesn't matter. There is no benefit in rushing through a dozen in fifteen minutes. Work steadily but perform each one carefully and with control. When the allotted time is up, save the rest of the routine for tomorrow. Varying your program day to day adds interest.

For those with neck problems, I've supplied several neck exercises. For those who wish to help lighten the burden on their backs, I've included some leg-strengthening exercises. These extra routines may be done alone or combined with the back exercises.

I encourage you to read the next section completely before making your decisions. Don't focus on just one or two items that sound useful; give yourself as much information as possible before you start.

For handy reference, I've also assembled the back exercises I outline into two easy-to-read charts. These are designed to provide at a glance suggested programs for all four types of back pain, both in the early stages of recovery and for long-term maintenance. They cover flexion and extension exercises, encompassing both stretching and strengthening routines.

EXERCISES FOR YOUR NECK, LEGS, AND BACK

Although the precise number of times you repeat a given exercise during each session may not make much difference in the long run, most of the exercises I describe here are intended for eight to ten repetitions each, unless my comments suggest otherwise.

Whatever number of repetitions you choose, take your time with them. You aren't in a race, and going slowly is not a matter of pampering yourself. In fact, it's more difficult, and therefore more beneficial, to do your exercises slowly than to repeat them as rapidly as you can, because speed can create that undesirable ballistic effect I mentioned earlier. The idea is *to provide gentle, controlled stretching and gradual strengthening while avoiding stress that may provoke pain*.

Most back patients who start to exercise worry about causing pain and wonder how much pain can be safely accepted. They should realize, however, that the pain caused by their original problem is not the same pain that comes from unaccustomed activity – that's a different sensation. Therapists at the Canadian Back Institute call it "sweet pain." It's a sensation I find impossible to define, but once you experience it I think you will agree "sweet" describes exactly the feeling of pain you know you can accept.

Neck Exercises

Strengthening the neck is just as important as strengthening the low back. In one respect, exercises for the neck are even more critical, because there are fewer passive ways you can protect your cervical spine. We have already discussed some easy ways to relieve stress on the lumbar area, such as standing with one foot raised on a rail or stool, or sitting with a pillow tucked into the small of your back – but there are no equivalent tricks you can use for your neck. Whether or not it remains free of pain depends almost entirely on the posture of your upper body and on the strength of the neck and shoulder muscles that support your head. That's a fact worth remembering when you are deciding whether to begin doing neck exercises regularly.

Ironically, one of the commonest causes of neck pain during exercise is the improper performance of low-back routines. When doing any flexion exercise for the low back, you should bring your neck and shoulders forward as a unit, keeping your chin tucked in. Straining with the neck to help lift the upper body puts unnecessary stress on the cervical spine and can lead to pain. It's been my experience that about two out of every ten patients who exercise for the low back report an increase of pain in their necks. It's almost always due to exercising improperly.

Stretching Exercises for the Neck and Shoulders

Neck Exercise 1: **THE SHRUG**

To start: Sit or stand in a relaxed manner.
The action: Raise your shoulders as high as you can. Hold that position to a slow count of eight. Then relax and pause before repeating.

Neck Exercise 2: **BACKWARD THRUSTING**

To start: Stand up or sit erect on a hard chair with your shoulders well clear of the chair back.
The action: With your arms loosely at your sides, thrust your shoulders as far back as they will go. Hold that position for a slow count of eight, then relax and pause before repeating.

Neck Exercise 3: **FORWARD THRUSTING**

To start: Stand up or sit erect on a hard chair with your shoulders well clear of the chair back.

The action: Thrust your shoulders forward as far as they will go. Hold that position for a slow count of eight, then relax before repeating.

Neck Exercise 4: **NECK ROTATION AND TILT**

To start: Stand or sit erect.

The action: Turn your head slowly to the left side and bring your chin down towards your shoulder as far as it will go. Return your head to the forward position. Now tip your head gently to the left as far as it will comfortably go, as if trying to place your ear on your shoulder, pause for one second, then return to the starting position. Repeat those two actions, alternating them and performing each one four times, working entirely to the left side. Now follow the same sequence to the right side.

Neck Exercise 5: **THE CHIN TUCK**

To start: Stand or sit erect.

The action: Keeping your head level, slowly tuck your chin in (not down) as far as possible. Keep staring straight ahead. Don't look up or down. Hold that position for a slow count of four, then relax before repeating.

Once you are comfortable with this exercise you can increase its effect by gently pushing on your chin with one hand after you have achieved your maximum tuck. Apply a gentle but firm degree of extra pressure.

Chin tucks can also be performed lying down as a method of relieving acute neck pain. Don't use a pillow. Lying on your back, slowly draw your chin in while you face the same spot on the ceiling to keep your head from tilting. Hold that position for a few seconds, then relax before repeating.

Strengthening Exercises for the Neck

These next four exercises pit one set of muscles against another. While they require a degree of firm pressure, you should *never* exert yourself to the point where your neck begins to quiver, since that movement will irritate the discs and facet joints in your cervical spine and probably cause pain. Once again, the key is moderation and slow, smooth movements.

Neck Exercise 6: **THE BACKWARD PRESS**

To start: Place your hands behind your head and clasp the fingers together securely.
The action: Tense your neck muscles by pushing your head back against your hands. Maintain the pressure to a slow count of eight. Relax before repeating.

Neck Exercise 7: **THE FORWARD PRESS**

To start: With your fingers pointing upwards, place the palms of your hands against your forehead.
The action: Press your head firmly forward against your hands to place tension on your neck muscles. Maintain the pressure to a slow count of eight. Relax before repeating.

Neck Exercise 8: **THE LEFT SIDE PRESS**

To start: With your fingers pointing upwards, place the palm of your left hand against the left side of your head just above your ear.
The action: Press your head firmly to the left against the hand. Hold this pressure through a slow count of eight. Relax before repeating.

Neck Exercise 9: **THE RIGHT SIDE PRESS**

To start: With your fingers pointing upwards, place the palm of your right hand against the right side of your head just above your ear.
The action: Same as for Exercise 8, but to the right instead.

Leg Exercises

In presenting exercises for your legs – principally to strengthen your thighs – I am not straying as far from the topic of back care as you might imagine. To protect your back from unnecessary strain, you need to use your legs as much as possible. Therefore, strong legs make for a healthy back.

Try these simple exercises to strengthen your legs:

Leg Exercise 1: **THE HALF KNEE BEND**

To start: Stand erect, with your feet comfortably apart, and place your hands on your hips.
The action: Keeping your feet flat on the floor, slowly bend your knees. Half way down, pause momentarily. Now straighten your knees slowly until you have returned to your starting position. Relax before repeating.

To get the most benefit from the half knee bend, perform it slowly and smoothly. If you descend quickly you are relying on gravity to lower your body instead of using your thigh muscles. By performing the movement in a controlled way, you introduce a constant muscular tension that builds the strength you need.

Leg Exercise 2: **THE IMAGINARY CHAIR**

To start: Stand with your back against a smooth wall, feet slightly apart and your arms at your sides.

The action: Press your back firmly against the wall and slide your body slowly downwards until your thighs are parallel to the floor. Don't move your feet forward; keep them directly below your knees. Don't press your hands onto the front of your thighs; that takes much of the load off your leg muscles. Hold this position as long as you can, then return slowly to your starting position.

This exercise is harder to do than it sounds. If you can remain seated in your imaginary chair for more than thirty seconds, you're doing well. Try a few seconds the first time and work up from there in subsequent sessions.

Back Exercises

As you will see, the back exercises I recommend here are separated into more than just flexion (forward bending) and extension (backward bending) routines. Each of these categories is divided, in turn, into exercises that stretch and others that strengthen. In all, there are four categories to choose from, according to your basic problem and your stage of improvement. The exercises that are best for you when you are recovering from an acute attack may need augmenting or replacing later on, when your trouble has healed and you are ready for a program of regular maintenance, as indicated by that designation in my comments on the application of each exercise.

If a particular exercise seems to increase your symptoms it's not right for you. For example, if you are Type Two, in an acute stage, a flexion exercise will probably cause pain. That simply means you are not ready for it. You should avoid flexion routines at that stage and try some other exercises recommended on my list. When the disc has healed you will be able to add forward bending (flexion) to your long-term program.

On the other hand, there is no need to progress automatically. If the first group of exercises you try makes your back feel better, stay with them and ignore the others. Sooner or later most people should gain additional flexibility, and if you feel you can handle some of the other exercises without pain, go ahead. But if they aggravate the situation, don't continue. The idea is not to do all the exercises but to find the ones that are right for you.

I recommend the same approach to the variations described for making individual strengthening exercises more difficult (and hence, for those who can do them, more rewarding). If the Level 1 version of a routine provides the relief you're looking for, don't feel that you must push on to Levels 2 and 3. Just count yourself lucky that you quickly found what you were looking for – and stay with it.

While it's often true, as you might assume, that the more strenuous exercises offer speedier improvement in your condition, they also pose a greater risk of discomfort or pain. And so, if you do decide to progress, protect yourself by adopting an increased amount of caution. Start the first routines of each session gently, avoiding violent and extreme movements. Just remember: while none of these routines will harm you, they can cause needless pain – and perhaps discourage you from continuing. Knowing when to do the various exercises is vital. You must gauge your progress carefully. As you will see in the comments on each exercise, some can be performed safely and usefully at "any time," while others are designated as suitable only "after recovery, for long-term maintenance," when your acute pain has resolved.

FLEXION (FORWARD BENDING) EXERCISES

Flexion exercises are designed both to strengthen the abdominal muscles that help support the back, and to increase flexibility by opening up the small joints along the spine while stretching the structures in the backs of the legs, notably the hamstring muscles. Traditionally it was believed that abdominal strengthening helped by increasing the body's ability to maintain a rigid column of air within the abdominal cavity. This column, often compared to a thick-walled balloon, becomes an additional support for the weight of the upper torso. A newer theory suggests that powerful belly muscles pull on strong fibrous sheets that encircle the trunk, creating tension near the spine and making the low back rigid and strong. Regardless of which theory is correct, strong abdominal muscles play an important part in reducing low-back pain.

Flexion exercises increase the load on the anterior column of the spine. If your pain is Type Two, that is from a disc, repeated flexion may increase your symptoms, and this type of exercise program should be stopped. If, however, the problem is primarily in the posterior column, that is Type One pain, you'll find flexion exercise routines lead to a gain in mobility and a decrease in discomfort. This is a subtle process, though, and you'll achieve your goal best if you go about these exercises gently.

For patients with resolving discogenic problems who are once again able to bend forward without pain, and are starting on a program that includes flexion exercises, the physical therapists at the CBI recommend alternating these exercises with equally strenuous extension maneuvers.

Strengthening the abdomen takes time, but it offers great rewards. As you do your flexion-strengthening exercises, you will notice that they require less and less effort and are associated with less and less back pain.

Performing some flexion-strengthening exercises incorrectly places extra stress on your neck and is a common cause of neck pain. Remember, you should bring your neck and shoulders forward as a single unit, keeping your chin tucked.

Flexion–Stretching

Back Exercise 1: **KNEES TO CHEST**

To start: Lie on your back in a crook position; that is, with your knees bent and your feet flat on the floor. Rest your arms at your sides. Adopt a pelvic tilt.
The action: Holding the pelvic tilt, draw both knees up to your chest. Maintain that position for a slow count of eight, and then return your legs to their original position. Relax before repeating.

Suitable for:
Type One – any time.
Type Two – after recovery, for long-term maintenance.
Type Three – after recovery, for long-term maintenance.
Type Four – any time.

This is an anti-gravity exercise designed to increase the flexibility of your spine and open up the facet joints.

If you have very weak abdominal muscles, try an easier version of this exercise by drawing up one bent knee at a time. The leg remaining on the floor helps steady the low back and maintains the pelvic tilt.

Back Exercise 2: ANKLE TOUCHING

To start: Sit on a chair and slump forward, with your feet on the floor, your knees bent, and your legs slightly spread.

The action: Bend forward slowly at the waist until your chest is on your knees. As you do, run your hands down the inside of your legs until you reach your ankles. Straighten up before repeating.

A more demanding variation: Instead of starting with your feet flat on the floor, extend your legs and rest your heels on the floor with your feet wide apart. This increases the pull on the back of your legs.

Suitable for:
Type One – any time.
Type Two – after recovery, for long-term maintenance.
Type Three – after recovery, for long-term maintenance.
Type Four – after recovery, for long-term maintenance.

Back Exercise 3: "TYING MY SHOE"

To start: Stand with one foot up on a low stool directly in front of you, with the straight leg bearing most of your weight.

The action: Bend forward until your chest touches the raised knee and your hands reach the raised foot.

Repeat this action four or five times, then reverse your position so that your other foot is on the stool.

Suitable for:
Type One – any time.
Type Two – after recovery, for long-term maintenance.
Type Three – after recovery, for long-term maintenance.
Type Four – after recovery, for long-term maintenance.

(continued on page 308)

Forward bending increases the load on the front of the spine, so proceed carefully. You may not be able to reach the final position in this exercise, but go as far as you can without producing a recurrence of your typical pain. By keeping one leg straight, you place tension on the nerves and muscles along the back of that leg. Keeping the other leg bent with your foot up on the stool reduces the pull on the rest of the back. If you have more stiffness or soreness in one leg, do a few extra repetitions with that leg straight, to help limber it up.

Back Exercise 4: **TOE TOUCHING**

To start: Stand with your legs straight but relaxed (not stiff), your feet comfortably apart, and your arms at your sides.
The action: Bend forward slowly at the waist, while allowing your arms to dangle loosely in front of you, until your upper body is horizontal and your back is slightly rounded. Now bring your trunk up again to the starting position. Relax before repeating.

Suitable for:
Type One – any time.
Type Two – after recovery, for long-term maintenance.
Type Three – after recovery, for long-term maintenance.
Type Four – after recovery, for long-term maintenance.

I always hesitate to recommend this exercise – not because it isn't good when done properly but because it is too often abused. I suggest you keep the following points in mind at all times:

  • Toe touching should *never* be done violently. While you are unlikely to damage yourself seriously, you may pull a muscle or cause other needless strain or pain.
  • You should not try to touch your toes while standing with your legs stiff and your feet together.
  • It doesn't really matter whether you actually touch your toes. The idea is simply to stretch the muscles and nerves in the low back and down the backs of your hips and legs.
  • The horizontal position should not be sustained. Straighten up as soon as you have felt a comfortable amount of stretch. People

with Type Two or Type Three pain must be particularly careful.

• Although the first few flexions may produce a little pain, the exercise should get easier and less painful with each repetition. Increasing discomfort means that toe touching should be discontinued.

Flexion–Strengthening

For some flexion-strengthening exercises, I define three levels of difficulty which depend on the position of your arms. Level 1 is the easiest position, Level 3 the hardest, and the progression from easy to difficult goes this way:

Level 1: arms extended over your legs.
Level 2: arms folded across your chest.
Level 3: hands over your ears, elbows out to the sides.

Note that in Level 3, the hands are *not* behind the head, since that position could allow you to pull your head forward and place unwanted stress on your neck.

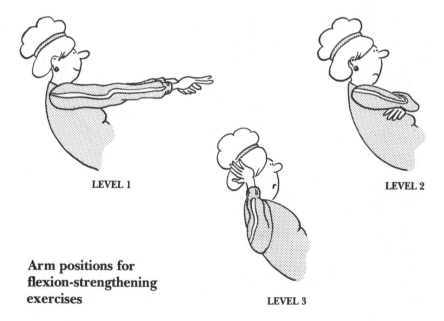

LEVEL 1

LEVEL 2

Arm positions for flexion-strengthening exercises

LEVEL 3

Back Exercise 5: **THE CROSS-OVER KNEE PUSH**

To start: Lie on your back in the crook position; that is, with your knees bent and your feet flat on the floor. Adopt a pelvic tilt: tighten your abdominal muscles and flatten the small of your back against the floor by rolling your hips forward and contracting the muscles in your buttocks. You can raise your buttocks slightly but do not push with your feet.

The action: Holding the pelvic tilt, bend your left knee and draw it toward your stomach. Keeping your arm straight, place your right hand on your left knee, raise your head and shoulders. Be sure to keep your chin tucked to avoid unwanted strain on your neck. Now use your right hand to push firmly on your left knee until you feel your abdominal muscles contracting. Hold the tension as you count slowly to eight. Relax momentarily and repeat the action four more times with the same arm and leg. Lower your left leg to the crook position, raise the right leg, and perform the pushing action with your left hand – counting, relaxing, and repeating as before.

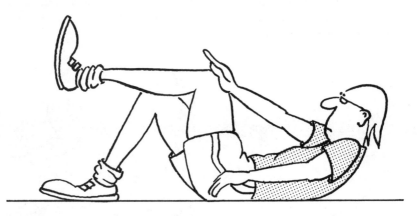

Suitable for:
Type One – any time.
Type Two – any time.
Type Three – after recovery, for long-term maintenance.
Type Four – any time.

Back Exercise 6: **THE ROLL-UP**

To start: Lie on your back in the crook position. Adopt a pelvic tilt. Tuck your chin to avoid neck strain.

The action: Holding the pelvic tilt, roll your body up, raising your head and shoulders forward and then bringing both knees up toward them. Now reverse the action, lowering your head and shoulders first, then your knees. Pause before repeating.

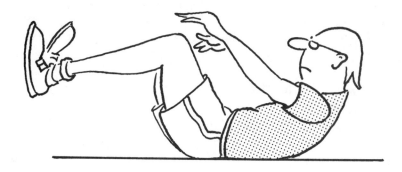

The roll-up can be done at any level:
Level 1: arms extended over your legs.
Level 2: arms folded across your chest.
Level 3: hands over your ears, elbows out to the sides.

Suitable for:
Type One – any time.
Type Two – after recovery, for long-term maintenance.

Back Exercise 7: **SUPINE LEG SPREADING**

To start: Lie on your back with both legs straight out on the floor. Adopt a pelvic tilt.

The action: Holding the pelvic tilt, bend both knees toward your chest, straighten your legs in the air, and lower them until they form a forty-five to sixty-degree angle with the floor. Now spread your legs apart and bring them back together eight times. Lower your legs. Relax before repeating. (continued on page 312)

Supine leg spreading can be attempted at three levels:
Level 1: arms extended over your legs.
Level 2: arms folded across your chest.
Level 3: hands over your ears, elbows out to the sides.

Suitable for:
Type One – after recovery, long-term maintenance.
Type Two – any time.
Type Three – after recovery, long-term maintenance.

The closer your legs are to the floor during this exercise the more difficult it becomes. Be careful not to lose your pelvic tilt.

Back Exercise 8: **THE SIT-UP**

To start: Lie on your back in the crook position. Adopt a pelvic tilt.
The action: Holding the pelvic tilt, raise your upper body slowly until your shoulder blades clear the floor. Hold that partly raised position to a slow count of eight. Lower yourself to the floor. Pause before repeating.

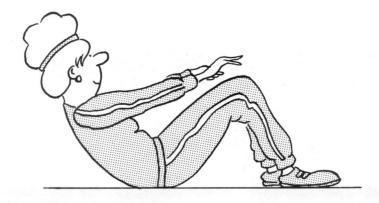

The sit-up can be attempted at three levels:
Level 1: arms extended over your legs.
Level 2: arms folded across your chest.
Level 3: hands over your ears, elbows out to the sides.

Suitable for:
Type One – any time.
Type Two – after recovery, long-term maintenance.
Type Three – after recovery, long-term maintenance.

Many people make the mistake of performing the sit-up starting with their legs straight out (or almost so) and their feet hooked under a piece of heavy furniture. That's not a bad exercise for your hips and thighs, but it doesn't help your belly muscles much. Electrical studies of muscular action have shown that with the legs held down, the action of bending at the waist takes place mainly by flexing the hips. With the feet free, the only way to perform the sit-up is to contract the stomach muscles. Keep your knees bent and try to hold your feet flat on the floor. Until you gain enough strength in your stomach you may notice that as you begin to raise your upper body your feet rise slightly in a counterbalancing action.

The sit-up is the ultimate exercise in its category. If you are going to do only one flexion-strengthening exercise, this is the one to do. Remember to keep your head and shoulders working as a unit. As you sit up, don't force your head forward or pull yourself up by putting your hands behind your neck. As I have already said, many people bring on neck pain by doing their low-back exercises incorrectly.

Another mistake people make with the sit-up is failing to sit up far enough. In a proper sit-up, your shoulder blades must completely clear the floor. Often people will raise their head and shoulders slightly, and then stop as soon as they feel tension. That's not enough. One way to guarantee that you sit up far enough is to lie on a mark made on the floor just above your waist. If someone watching you can see the mark under your body, you know you've risen far enough.

Many people complete their sit-ups to a full upright position. I don't believe there is anything wrong with this, although some physical therapists worry that it may increase the disc load unnecessarily. One thing we do agree on is that the final thirty degrees or so of elevation is easy to achieve, so, in fact, this last part of the full sit-up adds little benefit and makes the whole exercise less efficient. If that is your style of sit-up, you can improve your efficiency by sitting back very slowly and maintaining a strong abdominal contraction all the way to the floor.

Back Exercise 8A: **THE SIT-DOWN**

To start: Sit on the floor, bring your knees up and hold them with your hands.
The action: Maintaining a grip on your knees, lean back gradually. When your arms are fully extended, use them to pull yourself towards your knees again. Pause before repeating.

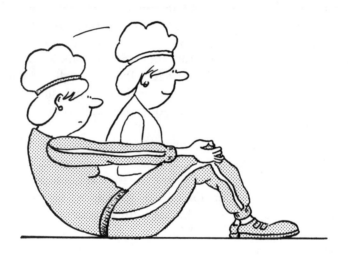

Suitable for:
Type One – any time.
Type Two – after recovery, for long-term maintenance.
Type Three – after recovery, for long-term maintenance.

This is the easiest sit-up of the three. It's a good way to get started if you find you have virtually no strength in your abdominal muscles, since your arms will provide the strength you need to sit up. Be patient; it can take months to develop your belly muscles. As they grow stronger, you'll find you can perform the sit-down by leaning back all the way to the floor and coming up again. Thus, with practice and increased muscle strength, the sit-down becomes the sit-up.

Back Exercise 8B: **THE BENCH SIT-UP**

To start: Lie on your back on the floor with your feet and the calves of your legs resting on the seat of a chair, sofa, or bench. If you're doing this correctly, your legs, thighs, and trunk will form a "z"; your thighs should be vertical and your lower legs parallel to the floor. Adopt a pelvic tilt.

The action: Holding the pelvic tilt, perform the sit-up as described, making sure your neck and shoulders move as a unit and your shoulder blades clear the floor. Pause and relax before repeating.

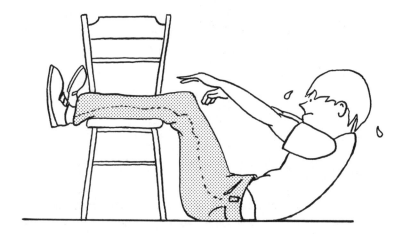

The bench sit-up can be attempted at three levels:

Level 1: arms extended over your legs.

Level 2: arms folded across your chest.

Level 3: hands over ears, elbows out to sides.

Suitable for:

Type One – any time.

Type Two – after recovery, for long-term maintenance.

The purpose of this variation is to further eliminate action of your thigh muscles, thereby placing an even greater load on the belly muscles themselves. It's the most difficult form of sit-up and is not for everyone. You should attempt it only if you're in generally good physical condition and find the standard sit-up lacking in challenge, even at Level 3.

EXTENSION EXERCISES

Extension exercises have two basic purposes. One is to strengthen the paraspinal muscles, located along your spine and felt as two ridges running down your back. The other is to increase flexibility by putting your facet joints through movements opposite to those done in forward bending. Because extension exercises increase the load on the facet joints they are usually uncomfortable for patients suffering from Type One pain.

For those suffering from a pinched nerve (Type Three) with significant leg pain, lying in extension can sometimes alter the location of the symptoms. The worst pain may shift from the leg into the back – an encouraging sign many physical therapists look for as an indication that the patient's condition is improving.

Extension–Stretching

Back Exercise 9: **PRONE LYING**

To start: Lie on your stomach. Put your hands together under your forehead. Turn your head to one side if you feel more comfortable that way.
The action: Lie there and count to ten. That's it – just lie there! Continue for as long as fifteen minutes at a stretch.

Suitable for:
Type One – after recovery, for long-term maintenance.
Type Two – any time.
Type Three – any time.
Type Four – as a possibility (see my comment below).

This one may sound like a heaven-sent instruction to some, and a real put-on to others, but it has its purpose: when you lie on your stomach, you automatically arch your back. And, as you may realize, that's exactly why this exercise is right for Type Two but unwise for Type One sufferers in the acute phase, when they typically can't arch their backs without pain.

Use any surface you find comfortable – a bed, a long couch, a well-carpeted floor; there is no advantage in choosing a hard surface (and no extra points for martyrdom). If you find this passive exercise position comforting, do it as often you like – while listening to the radio or conversing with visiting friends who are prepared to accept your eccentricities.

Most people with Type Four pain (spinal stenosis) do better on flexion-stretching routines, but a few find extension-stretching more helpful. I don't routinely recommend extension exercises for Type Four pain, but if that's your trouble, and you haven't been able to obtain benefit from flexion-stretching, you might try some extension-stretching and see what it does for you.

Back Exercise 10: **RESTING ON YOUR ELBOWS**

To start: Lie on your stomach and prop yourself up on your elbows.
The action: Hold that position at least to a slow count of ten – or for as long as you feel comfortable.

Suitable for:
Type One – after recovery, for long-term maintenance.
Type Two – any time.
Type Three – any time.
Type Four – as a possibility (see comment under Exercise 9).

This position, popular with children while watching television, is obviously just a variation of Exercise 9, but it increases the extension effect. My comments there also apply here.

Back Exercise 11: **THE "SEA LION" PUSH-UP**

To start: Lie on your stomach on a firm surface, with your forehead on the floor, your palms down, and your hands beside your shoulders.
The action: Gradually push yourself up with your hands and arms, raising your trunk from the waist up, while the rest of your body and your legs remain on the floor. Hold for a count of eight and then slowly lower your body again. Pause before repeating.

(continued on page 318)

Suitable for:
Type Two – any time.
Type Three – any time.

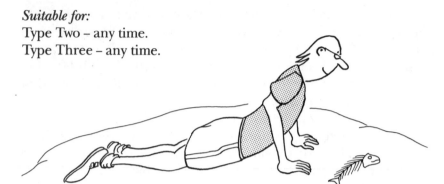

This may be the closest you ever come to looking like a sea lion sunning itself on a rock. Like the two previous exercises, this one will seem mild to anybody used to heavy workouts, but it's an active method of putting your spine through a full range of extension without straining your back muscles.

Back Exercise 12: **ARCHING BACKWARDS**

To start: Stand erect with feet comfortably apart and your hands on the small of your back.
The action: Gently arch backwards to look up· at the ceiling. Try not to bend your knees. Maintain this position for a count of eight. Pause before repeating.

Suitable for:
Type One – after recovery, for long-term maintenance.
Type Two – any time.
Type Three – after recovery, for long-term maintenance.
Type Four – as a possibility (see comment under Exercise 9).

As you will probably notice, this exercise is the action you have often performed instinctively whenever you stand up to stretch after sitting for a long time. As with flexion-stretching, you should perform this movement to the point of resistance – and then just a little more.

Like the flexion-stretching exercises, this movement should become increasingly easy for you with repetition and certainly not more painful. You should become gradually aware of an increased mobility. Moving any stiff joint will be painful at first, and it's important to assess the change in pain rather than simply reacting to that first twinge. If you don't feel any benefit after several sessions, try another exercise on the list.

Extension–Strengthening

As I did with the flexion-strengthening exercises, I have provided three levels of difficulty for some extension-strengthening exercises, as determined by the position of the hands. With extensions the hand positions are roughly the reverse of what they were for the flexion exercises. Level 1 is still the easiest, and Level 3 the most difficult:

Level 1: hands clasped behind the small of your back.
Level 2: hands clasped behind your neck.
Level 3: arms extended over your head.

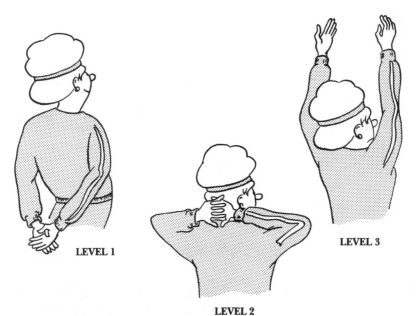

LEVEL 1

LEVEL 3

LEVEL 2

Arm positions for extension-strengthening exercises

Back Exercise 13: **HIP EXTENSION**

To start: Lie on your stomach. Put your hands together under your forehead. Turn your head to one side if you feel more comfortable that way.

The action: Bend one knee to a right angle, then, keeping that position, raise the front of the thigh off the floor. Hold the leg in the air for a slow count of eight. Repeat four times, then switch to the other leg and follow the same procedure.

A more demanding variation: Instead of bending your leg, keep it straight and lift from the hip. By extending your leg you create a longer lever, which makes the exercise more difficult.

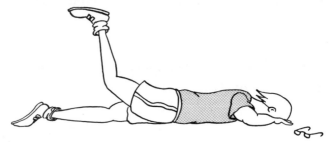

Suitable for:
Type One – after recovery, for long-term maintenance.
Type Two – any time.
Type Three – after recovery, for long-term maintenance.

Extending your hip (moving it backward) causes the paraspinal muscles to tense. Repeated movement strengthens not only the muscles of the buttocks, which are the principal hip extensors, but also the muscles along your spine.

Back Exercise 14: **TRUNK EXTENSION**

To start: Lie on your stomach with your hands clasped behind the small of your back.

The action: Tuck your chin, then slowly raise your head and chest until they clear the floor. Hold them up for a count of eight. Now lower them gently, then pause and relax before repeating.

Trunk extensions should be started at the first level of difficulty but can be done at all three levels:

Level 1: hands clasped behind the small of your back.
Level 2: hands clasped behind your neck.
Level 3: arms extended over your head.

Suitable for:
Type One – after recovery, for long-term maintenance; arm position at Level 1 only.
Type Two – any time.
Type Three – after recovery, for long-term maintenance.

Back Exercise 15: **TRUNK AND LEG RAISING**

To start: Lie on your stomach and bend your knees.
Clasp your hands behind the small of your back.
The action: Tuck your chin and then raise your head and upper torso slowly while lifting both legs until your thighs clear the floor. Hold for a slow count of eight. Pause and relax before repeating.

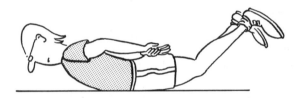

All three levels of difficulty are physiologically possible, but few people can manage Level 3 (arms over head), and even fewer should try. The three levels, again, are:
Level 1: hands clasped behind the small of your back.
Level 2: hands clasped behind your neck.
Level 3: arms extended over your head.

Suitable for:
Type Two – any time.

You can make this exercise even more difficult by keeping your legs straight as you lift them from the hips.

No one with Type One, Type Three, or Type Four pain should attempt this exercise; Type Two should use it carefully.

Back Exercise 16: **THE HORIZONTAL LIFT**

To start: Lie face down on a firm bed or table, with your lower body and legs on the surface and your upper body hanging, head down, over the edge.

The action: With a companion holding your legs down, raise your upper torso until your whole body is extended straight out. Hold the position for a slow count of eight, then slowly lower your body. Pause before repeating.

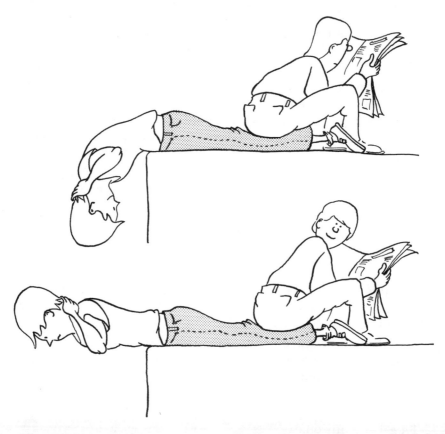

The horizontal lift can be done at any of the three levels of difficulty:

Level 1: hands clasped behind the small of your back.

Level 2: hands clasped behind your neck.

Level 3: arms extended over your head.

Suitable for:

Type One – after recovery, for long-term maintenance.
Type Two – after recovery, for long-term maintenance.
Type Three – after recovery, for long-term maintenance.

Just as the sit-up is the best flexion exercise for strengthening your abdomen, The Horizontal Lift is the best extension exercise for strengthening the paraspinal muscles. Lifting the weight of your upper body provides a real challenge.

Another advantage of this exercise is that it strengthens without requiring you to over-extend, since you are moving only from a forward-bent position up to neutral. This is especially helpful for Type One victims because they can develop their back muscles and still avoid forcing their facet joints into a painful, compressed position.

DR. HAMILTON HALL'S BACK EXERCISE CHART NO. 1
FOR THE RECOVERING PATIENT WHO IS JUST GETTING STARTED

TYPE OF PAIN	FLEXION (forward bending)		EXTENSION (backward bending)	
	Stretching Exercise	Strengthening Exercise	Stretching Exercise	Strengthening Exercise
Type 1	1. Knees to Chest 2. Ankle Touching 3. "Tying My Shoe" 4. Toe Touching	5. The Cross-Over Knee Push 6. The Roll-Up 8. The Sit-Up 8A. The Sit-Down 8B. The Bench Sit-Up	None	None
Type 2	None	5. The Cross-Over Knee Push 7. Supine Leg Spreading	9. Prone Lying 10. Resting on Your Elbows 11. The "Sea-Lion" Push-Up 12. Arching Backwards	13. Hip Extension 14. Trunk Extension 15. Trunk and Leg Raising
Type 3	None	None	9. Prone Lying 10. Resting on Your Elbows 11. The "Sea Lion" Push-Up	None
Type 4	1. Knees to Chest 2. Ankle Touching	5. The Cross-Over Knee Push	9. Prone Lying* 10. Resting on Your Elbows* 12. Arching Backwards *as possibilities see pp. 316-317	None

DR. HAMILTON HALL'S BACK EXERCISE CHART NO. 2
LONG-TERM CHOICES FOR KEEPING IN SHAPE

TYPE OF PAIN	FLEXION (forward bending)		EXTENSION (backward bending)	
	Stretching Exercise	Strengthening Exercise	Stretching Exercise	Strengthening Exercise
Type 1	1. Knees to Chest 2. Ankle Touching 3. "Tying My Shoe" 4. Toe Touching	5. The Cross-Over Knee Push 6. The Roll-Up 7. Supine Leg Spreading 8. The Sit-Up 8A. The Sit-Down 8B. The Bench Sit-Up	9. Prone Lying 10. Resting on Your Elbows 12. Arching Backwards	13. Hip Extension 14. Trunk Extension (Level 1 only) 16. The Horizontal Lift
Type 2	1. Knees to Chest 2. Ankle Touching 3. "Tying My Shoe" 4. Toe Touching	5. The Cross-Over Knee Push 6. The Roll-Up 7. Supine Leg Spreading 8. The Sit-Up 8A. The Sit-Down 8B. The Bench Sit-Up	9. Prone Lying 10. Resting on Your Elbows 11. The "Sea Lion" Push-Up 12. Arching Backwards	13. Hip Extension 14. Trunk Extension 15. Trunk and Leg Raising 16. The Horizontal Lift
Type 3	1. Knees to Chest 2. Ankle Touching 3. "Tying My Shoe" 4. Toe Touching	5. The Cross-Over Knee Push 7. Supine Leg-Spreading 8. The Sit-Up 8A. The Sit-Down	9. Prone Lying 10. Resting on Your Elbows 11. The "Sea Lion" Push-Up 12. Arching Backwards	13. Hip Extension 14. Trunk Extension 16. The Horizontal Lift
Type 4	1. Knees to Chest 2. Ankle Touching 3. "Tying My Shoe" 4. Toe Touching	5. The Cross-Over Knee Push	9. Prone Lying* 10. Resting on Your Elbows* 12. Arching Backwards *as possibilities see pp. 316-317	None

INDEX

Page numbers for illustrations are in italics.